THE BEAUTY OF
DIRTY SKIN

THE BEAUTY OF

DIRTY SKIN

The Surprising Science to Looking and Feeling Radiant from the Inside Out

Whitney Bowe, MD

with Kristin Loberg

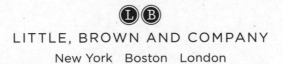

LITTLE, BROWN AND COMPANY

New York Boston London

Little, Brown and Company
Hachette Book Group
1290 Avenue of the Americas, New York, NY 10104
littlebrown.com

First Edition: April 2018

Little, Brown and Company is a division of Hachette Book Group, Inc.
The Little, Brown name and logo are trademarks of Hachette Book Group, Inc.

The publisher is not responsible for websites (or their content) that are not owned by the publisher.

The Hachette Speakers Bureau provides a wide range of authors for speaking events. To find out more, go to hachettespeakersbureau.com or call (866) 376-6591.

ISBN 978-0-316-50982-4
LCCN 2017959143

10 9 8 7 6 5 4 3

LSC-C

Printed in the United States of America

This book is dedicated to the loves of my life — my tiny angel,
Maclane, and my wonderful husband, Josh. Maclane, may you
continue to glow from within and light up the world the way
you light up my heart! And Josh, your support, love, and
fierce belief in me and my dreams make me the luckiest wife;
I could not love and adore you more.

Contents

INTRODUCTION: Learning to Love Your Good Bugs   3

PART I
A GUT REACTION TO RADIANT SKIN

CHAPTER 1   Nature's Hidden Secret to Great Skin   21
Why Getting Clear, Glowing Skin Is an Inside Job

CHAPTER 2   The New Science of Skin   48
Understanding the Gut-Brain-Skin Connection

CHAPTER 3   Mind over Skin Matters   63
The Brain's Influence on the Body, Inside and Out

CHAPTER 4   Face Value   77
What You Know About Skin Care Is Wrong

CHAPTER 5   The Power in Going Pro   91
Why Probiotics Are the New Antibiotics

PART II
GLOW WITH YOUR GUT

CHAPTER 6   Feed Your Face   113
Dietary Recommendations for Putting Your
Best Face Forward

CHAPTER 7   Take Time to Recover   143
The Power of Exercise, Meditation, and Sleep

Contents

CHAPTER 8   Handle with Care   160
*Reassess Your Regimen and Commit Daily to
Proper Skin Care*

CHAPTER 9   Supercharge Your Skin   185
Navigating the Supplements and Probiotics Aisle

PART III
PUTTING IT ALL TOGETHER

CHAPTER 10   Three Weeks to Radiant   203
Your Plan of Action for Smooth, Youthful, Clear Skin

CHAPTER 11   Recipes   234
Meals and Masks to Get Your Bowe Glow On

ACKNOWLEDGMENTS   249
NOTES   253
INDEX   267

THE BEAUTY OF
DIRTY SKIN

Introduction

Learning to Love Your Good Bugs

As a kid, I was always covered in dirt. I loved to dig in the earth, and I loved frogs and grass and bugs. Once, I even hid a snake in my overalls, which caused quite a stir when my kindergarten teacher discovered it! I was a blond-haired, blue-eyed, rosy-cheeked free spirit who dirtied a set of clothes about as fast as I could change into them. But that was all before I got sick.

You see, that carefree little girl spent her tenth year of life in and out of the hospital. The environment was sterile and cold. I was afraid. I was in pain—awful, chronic pain. The doctors didn't know how to help me. My parents didn't know how to help me, either.

It turns out that a bad bug—a parasite—had made its way into my intestines from fish I had eaten while on a family vacation. It wreaked complete havoc on my body. Even worse, the doctors couldn't find it. They tried to treat me with antibiotic after antibiotic, which eventually destroyed the healthy bacteria in my gut, leaving behind an infectious type of bad bacteria called *Clostridium difficile,* or C. diff, which made me even sicker. This horrific combination of circumstances, in which one bad microbe was followed by another, hurt my body and changed my life.

But all was not lost, because as I sat in the hospital, I started to think. Even as a ten-year-old, I could reason, explore, ask questions, and try

3

to make sense of things (maybe it was my way of coping). I knew that where we have bad, we always have good. It's the age-old balance between good and evil. So where we have harmful microbes, we also have helpful microbes—although the beneficial ones that had been slaughtered in my gut by antibiotics could no longer help me. This thinking process is where the happy ending to my story began—it started me on a passionate lifelong quest to find the answers to the question of how to create and maintain a balance between the heroic and villainous microbes that live in our bodies and on our skin.

From the moment I was released from the hospital, I was inspired to make my body strong and healthy. I was concerned with the obvious outward signs of health, such as glowing, radiant skin, as well as the hidden, invisible indicators of health, the ones that lie deep beneath the surface. This is where my passion for health and beauty from the outside in and the inside out was born. And this is where my fascination with the science of the microbial bugs that exist on our skin and throughout our bodies, including in our gut, initially began, because I experienced this balance (or imbalance) firsthand. Who better to investigate the depths of this area of science than someone who fought for her life because of it?

I succeeded in what I set out to achieve: a robust body that emanates health. Now I help others achieve that goal. In so many ways, I am still that happy and curious rosy-cheeked girl who loves nature. But now I'm also a doctor who has found a lot of answers to those lifelong questions. My curiosity about microbiology has only grown fiercer now that science is finally grasping the magnitude of the influence that the hidden microbial world within us—and on us—has over our health. And this dazzling new science shows definitively that these invisible bugs have a lot to do with how we look. I now know, as you're about to learn, that even on my best day, I have microorganisms in the form of bacteria, fungi, viruses, and even mites living all over my body that support my health from the inside out and give me that "Bowe Glow." And even on your best day, you're a "dirty" human being, too, whose health and appearance hinges on those bugs! (And if you're not having your best day now, read on.)

Learning to harness those things that make you "dirty" will help you radiate a healthy, beautiful glow from the outside in and the inside out. Your skin is a window on your overall health. It "speaks" to the other integral parts of your body through something called the gut-brain-skin axis, a pathway that you will get to know and understand in these pages. This groundbreaking science has become my life's work and has earned me recognition among my colleagues and among international thought leaders. Now let's take an expedition together to find *your* most luminous skin and overall wellness using the best cutting-edge science and tools available today. Like me, you'll learn to love your good bugs and harness your body's full potential. Let's show that ten-year-old little girl in the hospital bed that the story turns out *beautifully!*

THE SECRET TO GREAT SKIN

Take a moment to think about your skin. Find a mirror, if that helps. How does your skin feel and look? How do you feel about it? What do you think it says about you? Think of your skin's appearance as a reflection of your overall health—how healthy do you look?

Within seconds of meeting a new patient, I can use my derm super-powers (well, years of extensive training and developing expertise, but that doesn't sound as cool) to determine her overall health simply by examining her skin, hair, and nails. Is she diabetic or prediabetic? Does she eat a Western diet laden with processed sugars and refined carbs? Is her life overscheduled and full of constant, unremitting stress? Does she suffer from obsessive-compulsive disorder? A dysfunctional thyroid?

An imbalanced hormonal system? An autoimmune disorder? Insomnia? Does she have a history of frequent antibiotic use, either orally or topically or both? Is she overly hygienic, scrubbing her skin with harsh cleansers and facial brushes? Is her gastrointestinal system in need of serious repair?

My patients come to me hoping to get the Bowe Glow. Too often, they believe they're just a scribbled prescription away from a cure for any of the Big Four—acne, rosacea, eczema, and premature aging. But there's so much more than drugs, topical lotions, or laser beams to this story. Every day I have the privilege of interacting with smart, health-conscious people who try to maintain their looks and health as best they can, but they often miss the mark because they don't have access to eye-opening knowledge that is still mostly buried in the trenches of scientific literature. But the good news is that with this book, I'm giving you access to this information and grounding it in my expertise and years of experience treating thousands of patients. And here's the secret: the road to a beautiful glow begins with simple lifestyle habits that support the **gut–brain–skin relationship**, which is the soul of radiant skin. More specifically, I'm referring to the bonds between the body's good bugs and the brain and skin.

You've probably heard about the human microbiome by now, but trying to fully understand it might still give you pause. Much has been written in the past few years about the microbiome—the friendly microorganisms that support our health and share a powerful, mutually beneficial relationship with our bodies. The term *microbiome* comes from the combination of *micro,* for "super small" or "microscopic," and *biome,* which refers to a naturally occurring community of life forms occupying a large habitat, in this case the human body. When I began to study microbiology as a junior-high-school student, nobody could tell you what a microbiome was; today, microbiology encompasses one of the hottest fields of study, and I'm proud to be a part of it. We are at the very beginning of an exciting journey to understanding—and leveraging the power of—the human microbiome.

The mini ecosystem that comprises a human biome includes a diverse collection of microorganisms, mainly bacteria, fungi, and viruses. The bacteria that thrive in our intestines are especially important. Their function in our health and physiology is so critical that they may affect a wide range of biological processes and play a role in everything from the efficiency and speed of our metabolism to our risk for diabetes and obesity. This is to say nothing of their potential role in our moods and our likelihood of suffering from depression, autoimmune disorders, and dementia. Perhaps you have heard about some of this in the popular health media. But there's another connection that you probably don't know about: the "last mile." This is the indelible, incredible link from the brain to the skin. Indeed, what's going on in your gut right at this moment is determining not only how your brain performs and responds to signals from the body about its current state and needs but also what your *skin* thinks and how it performs. This gut-brain-skin alliance is, frankly, profound and breathtaking, as this book will show. And yes, the skin can "think" and "talk" to the brain: it's a two-way street. In fact your skin actually contains the same number of cells as sixteen human brains!

Your Skin Has Company

The skin of an average adult can be spread across a twenty-two-square-foot room. There are more than one trillion bacteria in your skin alone, coming from around one thousand different species. All these microbial living creatures are part of your skin's health and behavior, and in some cases they provide vital functions for the skin that the human body cannot perform all on its own. If your skin's ecosystem is off balance, you can experience any number of skin conditions.

Researchers first discovered this relationship more than one hundred years ago, but it was forgotten until recently. Today the gut-brain-skin axis is among the most thought-provoking areas of study, and I believe it represents a revolution in our field—not least because it equips us dermatologists with a breakthrough approach to the way we think about the skin. For the first time, we can envision a future in which we aren't just chasing skin issues that are spiraling out of control, we're also finding ways to get to the root of the problem. We're stopping the proverbial match from being lit in the first place.

I played a major role in rediscovering this link, having spent years in the lab counting bacterial colonies in a petri dish whenever I wasn't poring through databases looking at epidemiological data to support my suspicions. I loved studying bacteria and figuring out what they could do—both to help us and harm us. By the time I'd chosen dermatology as a specialty, I was determined to make the connection between the secret world of microscopic bugs and the outer world of skin's appearance. Which bugs could benefit skin health? Which could harm it? I even coinvented a patented acne treatment that uses a substance isolated from a certain bacterium. This patent was filed through the University of Pennsylvania with my research mentor, Dr. David Margolis. That's right: we can now use good bacteria to fight bad bacteria in the battle against acne, which can be driven by a particular strain of bacteria. I've shared my research and theories with my peers internationally through numerous scientific publications and lectures. And in 2017, I was humbled to receive the American Academy of Dermatology's presidential citation for this work.

Too many people suffer in silence with their skin conditions because they lack access to the kind of information I am going to provide in this book. I can only reach so many individuals in my private practice, many of whom are in the public eye daily. Their livelihoods depend on looking good, but they shouldn't be the only ones fortunate enough to have flawless skin. With this book, I bring hope, health, and beauty to as many people as possible. That means *you*, no matter what you do for a living or where you live.

SKIN TELLS THE TRUTH: YOU ARE WHAT YOU EAT

You might be surprised to find that food is at the core of my program. But don't panic: I won't ask you to do anything drastic like totally give up chocolate, alcohol, bread, or coffee if those things bring you joy. I trust you'll find the dietary protocol outlined in chapter 6 to be refreshingly delicious, inspiring, inviting, and, above all, doable.

Contrary to long-held beliefs in my field, diet, first and foremost, determines the quality and appearance of your skin. Food provides information for every cell that makes you, well, *you*. Everything you eat becomes part of not only your inner cellular makeup but also the outer fabric of your body. In fact there's no more direct way to change the health of your body's inner and outer ecology — its microbiome — than to make specific shifts in your dietary choices. Yes, this probably goes against everything you've been told about the relationship between diet and skin. Have no doubt. The idea that food is arguably the most important factor in personal health, including the health of your skin, is old news gaining new life in our modern medical world.

When I was in medical school, and even during my residency training in dermatology, we were taught that diet had no impact on the skin. All the major dermatology textbooks stated that the exception was in cases of severe malnutrition, which were exceedingly rare in developed countries such as the United States. Textbooks, lectures, and reputable authorities such as the American Academy of Dermatology told us that if a patient suggested that what she was eating or drinking had any influence on her skin, we were to dismiss that notion as a myth. This was the scientific dogma of the time, and it was based on research conducted and published by physicians who were revered as giants and geniuses in our area.

But what I was experiencing with my own skin, and what I observed in my patients, didn't seem to fit with this alleged fact. So I approached my mentor, who also happened to be the chairman of the department at the time, and I presented him with my skepticism. Looking back, I can't believe I was bold (crazy?) enough to think that I, a young resident in training with barely any real experience under my belt, could take on such a monumental challenge. But I couldn't ignore what my body was telling me and what my patients were sharing with me every day.

My mentor advised me that if I was going to question the word of these highly respected authorities—lionized experts, really—in my field, I had better develop an incredibly compelling argument to support my theory. With a rebellious spark in my belly, I went back to the peer-reviewed scientific literature and dug deep, reading journals from all fields of medicine and nutrition and going so far as to have several international studies translated into English. I mined the few studies published in the late 1970s that were often cited as proof that diet had no impact on the skin, and I carefully dissected them, finding major flaws in their design. In fact if judged against the rigorous criteria by which journal submissions are considered today, these articles would never even have been published!

After many long days and late nights, I wrote a controversial paper that asserted the idea that diet does indeed affect the skin.[1] Armed with compelling evidence, I laid out the case that acne is exacerbated by diets loaded with sugar and refined carbohydrates. I also called out the fact that some dairy products trigger acne, and I hinted at the positive effects of omega-3 fatty acids and dietary fiber. Ultimately my paper was published in one of my field's most respected journals, heralding a new era for understanding skin health within the context of diet. And my mission didn't end there. I took to the lectern, speaking again and again on this topic, and over the years I published even more studies further supporting my hypothesis—a belief that was soon becoming indisputable fact. Although most of my peers were initially skeptical, as any good doctor should be when presented with new and competing data, I found increasingly that my dermatology audience was receptive to my message. Eventually other thought leaders emerged, contributing to the literature and spreading their own observations and research on how certain foods and beverages affect the skin. The data only grew bigger and more extensive and impressive. No one could turn me and my ideas down anymore.

Finally, for the first time since the late 1970s, dermatological textbooks, resources, and guidelines are being revised to reflect this concept. If a patient goes to her dermatologist with a hunch that certain foods are making her skin condition worse, not only can the dermatologist acknowledge that she is probably right, the doctor can also go so far as to offer evidence-based advice on how the patient can tweak her diet to benefit her skin (less sugar, milk, and processed foods; more fibrous, colorful vegetables, fatty fish, and antioxidant-rich fruits). I'm thrilled not only that my peers have accepted this concept as fact but also that laypersons and media are listening with open ears. This "new" fact could not have emerged at a more critical time.

WELCOME TO A NEW ERA

The field of dermatology is changing radically as a result of two immense forces: an epidemic of skin disorders in a world where powerful drugs such as antibiotics are losing their efficacy, and new findings about the power of the microbiome on skin health (and all health, really). Skin issues are the cause of more than 42 percent of all doctor visits.[2] No doubt this staggering statistic is largely attributable to the fact that you can't hide from your skin. You wear your illness for the world to see, and unless you're going to cover yourself up indefinitely or refuse to leave the house (two impractical, depressing prospects), you're going to seek help. Such conspicuous imperfections can have a colossal impact on one's overall mental health and sense of self.

I can't tell you how many times I've heard stories from people who breezed through their teenage and young adult lives pimple-free only to meet angry red spots and lumps covering their chins and faces in their thirties and forties. Acne has long been viewed as a rite of passage through adolescence, but it's not something an adult should be grappling with. What's going on? A whopping 54 percent of women age twenty-five and over have at least one type of facial acne.[3] And other skin disorders are on the rise, including the scariest one of all: skin cancer. In 2017, a report by the Mayo Clinic sent shock waves through the medical community, stating that between 2000 and 2010, squamous cell carcinoma (also called cutaneous squamous cell carcinoma) diagnoses increased 263 percent, while diagnoses of basal cell carcinomas increased 145 percent.[4] These numbers are mind-boggling given the level of sunscreen use today. To say we're entering a new era of skin conditions is an understatement. We're also embarking on new treatment territory, and I'll be discussing all this in the pages that follow.

Dermatologists only make up 1 percent or less of all doctors, but we prescribe almost 5 percent (if not more) of all antibiotics, which have long been held as the gold standard for treating many skin conditions.[5] Now, in the wake of rising antibiotic resistance, we are forced to look elsewhere for solutions. Part of my work today involves passionate formal talks to other dermatologists and doctors about this dire matter and pushing for change. I am sounding the alarm. We dermatologists are part of the problem, but we need to be part of the solution. The silver lining of the antibiotic crisis, however, is that it's opening the door to understanding the power of balanced gut microbes and probiotics in the treatment of skin. As the term suggests, probiotics (meaning "for life") are beneficial strains of live bacteria that you can ingest through foods, some beverages, and supplements. The science in this area is exploding with new research to show that probiotics can help recolonize the intestinal microbiome and can even help balance certain hormones. We'll be exploring all these mechanisms, which have everything to do with skin health. The science behind topically applied probiotics is also a burgeoning area of study. We'll see how your skin's microbiome has a big say in your skin's health and function.

Some of the information in this book will serve as a wake-up call you did not expect. Get ready to ditch a few of your trusty daily habits and establish new, unexpected ones. Do you drink milk and diet soda? Time to rethink. Do you go through the same physical exercise routine almost every day? Or barely bust a move at all and have no personal downtime? Time to rethink. Do you use hand sanitizers and anti-microbial soaps, or regularly wash your face with exfoliating scrubs or tools like brushes, loofahs, and abrasive washcloths? Time to reassess. But again, don't worry about bracing for extreme overnight changes. I promise to make this practical for the real world. Hey, I still love to play outside under the sun and eat pancakes on Sundays. And yes, I have been known to get fully dressed in workout clothes only to climb back into bed with my daughter and wake up an hour later when it's time to get her dressed for school. I'm not your typical dermatologist, one who preaches staying in the shade. I want my patients and readers to live out loud and feel their most confident every single day. To find that balance we all seek in life. To cherish their health and to make the most of it.

Most dermatologists, for example, will tell rosacea patients to avoid typical triggers. Want to know what those are? Exercise, alcohol, hot beverages, spicy foods, hot temperatures, and very cold temperatures.

From my perspective, that's like asking someone to zap all the joy out of life (and it's no wonder patients with rosacea have a hard time being compliant with those recommendations). Unrealistic. What kind of life is there without a margarita and Mexican food once in a while? How can I expect someone to start her day without a hot cup of joe? And how could I possibly tell someone not to exercise when we know how much exercise benefits the entire body? Yes, there are certain things that can trigger certain skin problems, but my goal is to find workable, real-life solutions so no one feels deprived.

You will *never* hear me ask my patients to give up all the things that make life fun and contribute to overall health and well-being for the sake of their skin. Moderation is key. I am all about finding ways to get these skin conditions under control while living life to the fullest and relishing every moment. My message is equally about self-empowerment, self-improvement, and liberation from the clutches of feeling unattractive. I know of no easier or quicker way to get more of what you want out of life than to first love the skin you're in, as the old Olay commercial advises.

In this book I present a revolutionary new way to think about and take care of your skin. Whether you're hoping to end a chronic skin condition or enhance your skin's appearance, you'll find easy, simple solutions you can implement in your life right away and see results relatively quickly—in as little as three weeks. No surgery or prescriptions are required. (Of course, it's fine if you are already following a course of treatment recommended by a dermatologist, and it's fine if you want to visit a dermatologist today and use my program in combination with a formally prescribed regimen. This program is super compatible with prescribed treatments.) Soon you will learn to love your good bugs and let your personal transformation unfold before your eyes.

This isn't just about skin, either. The strategies in this book will elevate everything about your health. Happy, glowing skin is a reflection of overall general health. And you'll gain other measurable benefits, such as

- weight loss,
- increased energy,
- better sleep and less insomnia,
- reduced stress and better coping mechanisms,
- relief from moodiness, anxiety, and depression,
- a reduction in gastrointestinal conditions, including chronic constipation and bloating,
- a lessening or reversal of metabolic disorders, including insulin resistance and diabetes,
- heightened mental clarity,
- a stronger immune system and reduced autoimmunity,
- a more youthful appearance,
- and more.

In the pages ahead, we're going to get up close and personal with this remarkable organ called skin. In part I, you'll learn more about why getting clear, glowing skin is an inside job—from your state of mind and how your gut functions to what you put in your mouth and on your skin. You'll gain a skin-care education that probably goes against conventional wisdom (be prepared to throw some of your beauty products away). Then, in part II, you'll learn practical tools that will transform you and your skin. By the time you reach my three-week action plan in part III, you'll be primed—and excited—to put these ideas into practice. You'll be making subtle, doable shifts in your daily habits, from what you eat for breakfast to how you exercise, reduce stress, supplement with vitamins and probiotics, ensure restful sleep, and treat your face.

Get ready to go. And get ready to *glow.*

PART I

A Gut Reaction to Radiant Skin

You are here because you want to know the secrets behind glowing, beautiful skin. I have dedicated my life's work to uncovering those secrets, and you're about to read about them. But they are not as "new" as you might think. While the science of great skin may seem like a subject that's in rapid development today, thanks to our burgeoning knowledge of the role of the human microbiome, we actually began to understand this information more than one hundred years ago. The difference, however, is that now we finally know how to leverage it for our skin's (and whole body's) benefit. It is no longer a mystery how exactly the gut, brain, and skin are all connected.

In this first part, we're going on a tour of the groundbreaking research from past to present and will even cast off to what lies ahead in the near future so you are prepared to benefit. I will share all this captivating information in an easy, accessible way that will have you making mental notes and rethinking how you're living each day. You will learn a wealth of useful, highly practical knowledge that will inspire you to execute my program right away. By the end of this part, you will have a new appreciation for the interconnectedness of your body's systems and parts, including its microbiome. It is now proved that your skin reflects your diet, sleep schedule, stress levels, exercise regimen, and of course the health of your microbiome. And, as you will soon experience, the power of glowing, healthy skin is so much more than skin deep. When you feel wonderful about your skin, you unlock your confidence, courage, and overall well-being. I am so excited to share this gift with you. Knowledge is not just power. It is your ticket to looking—and feeling—beautiful. Your glow starts here.

CHAPTER 1

Nature's Hidden Secret to Great Skin

Why Getting Clear, Glowing Skin Is an Inside Job

You know it when you see it. The woman who walks into a room and attracts everyone's notice. A gravitational force surrounds her presence — a je ne sais quoi that makes her beautiful. But her beauty transcends physicality. Something about this individual speaks compellingly to others as she radiates health, grace, strength, vitality, and confidence. Her glowing skin reflects this all-encompassing sense of wellness. And she is living life to the fullest.

You're reading these pages for a reason. You've made a choice to take better care of yourself. With the plan in this book, you'll learn how to do so in a way that helps you achieve the smoothest, clearest, most beautiful skin possible. As a result, you, too, can become the best version of yourself. More self-assured. More outgoing and adventurous. Even more successful, too. Somewhere deep down you know that there's a hidden power to having great skin. And you're right.

From my vantage point as someone who helps people cultivate gorgeous skin, I don't need a scientific study to tell me how transformative satisfaction in one's appearance can be. You know that when you love your looks, anything is possible. But what you might not know is how much of an "inside job" getting that great skin is and how much it reflects overall wellness. Let me share with you some little-known facts to prepare you for your journey to healthier skin and a healthier body, starting with some alarming statistics. This, my friends, will help you see that you're not alone.

If you're suffering from a skin condition, you're among the majority. Tens of millions of people in the United States live with chronic skin conditions, which have been on a steep rise in the last two decades—right alongside autoimmune and other chronic diseases not caused by a germ or pathogen. Sixty million Americans, including adults, have acne (an estimated 85 percent of us have acne at some point).[1] Thirty-five million suffer from eczema, also called atopic dermatitis, a chronic condition that causes the skin to become itchy, red, dry, and cracked. Psoriasis, another chronic but autoimmune-based skin ailment, affects 7.5 million Americans. And at least sixteen million have rosacea, which is common in adults and is characterized by redness and visible blood vessels in the face. There are more than three thousand diseases of the skin treated by dermatologists. These numbers are so large as to seem meaningless. Most of us can get through life without being diagnosed with a rare illness, but none of us reaches adulthood without at least one skin affliction, be it a pimple, rash, superficial burn, or sunburn (one in five Americans will develop skin cancer over the course of a lifetime, largely because of overexposure to the sun). And nobody escapes the march of time in the form of aging, whether it's gradual and natural or fast and premature (as in, *Where did that line come from? What's happening to me?!*).

As a dermatologist who juggles the competing demands of lecturing to peers, treating patients, and appearing in the media regularly to talk about matters involving skin and the outward signs of aging, I try to keep abreast of all the latest and greatest when it comes to addressing skin disorders. Never has there been a more thrilling time in dermatology: we are experiencing a rapid expansion of our understanding of skin, its properties, and its connection to the rest of the body. The fact that I can detect a wide variety of illnesses by looking at a person's skin says a lot about the interconnectedness of the human body, from its deepest recesses to its outermost layer. I've identified an untold number of afflictions in patients who have come to me about a seemingly isolated topical skin issue. These afflictions include lupus, thyroid disease, certain cancers (including lung cancer), congenital heart disease and birth defects of the heart, peripheral artery disease, chronic obstructive pulmonary disease (COPD, or emphysema), cirrhosis (liver disease), anemia, alcoholism, Cushing's syndrome, Addison's disease, polycystic ovary syndrome, diabetes, and lymphoma. Indeed, the skin is not a solitary, secluded organ that works all on its own. It's highly dependent upon what's going on in remote areas of your body, where the sun doesn't shine.

My patients have taught me so much over the years. Their conditions are just a very small piece of who they are. I pour my heart and soul into working with them and helping them to look and feel their most empowered. It is very much a team effort. As I mentioned in the introduction, during my early days of training, I routinely saw a disconnect between what I was learning from my textbooks and lectures and what I saw and experienced firsthand—both in regard to my own body and my patients' signs and symptoms. Thank goodness I listened intently to my patients and followed my gut instincts!

Nowadays, you get to choose how fast you age, whether you prefer to use at-home protocols combined with affordable drugstore products or go the route of my celebrity patients who use cutting-edge in-office procedures in combination with a sophisticated daily skin-care regimen. How can I say this with confidence? Because every day I witness the transformation in my patients, many of whom are dealing with very stubborn skin disorders. And many of them begin to see major changes through highly practical strategies anyone can implement. They simply work from the inside out, healing those innermost, hidden corners of their bodies in order to generate radiance.

WHEN LIFESTYLE HABITS AFFECT SKIN

I always look forward to my appointments with Jennifer. She is one of those high-energy types with a magnetic presence, colorful both in her personality and in her amazing fashion picks! With a knack for being acutely aware of the next big trends in beauty, makeup, and hair, she is often into something fresh and new that she likes to talk about when I see her. I had been working with Jennifer for about six months to treat her rosacea. Through a series of laser treatments, dietary changes, and stress management strategies, we had gotten her skin condition beautifully under control, and her skin had looked fantastic at our last appointment. Happy patient, happy doctor!

I was definitely surprised and concerned when, at a follow-up appointment, I went into the exam room to find that her rosacea was not only back but had also flared up substantially. Something was going on, and we needed to get to the bottom of it.

Jennifer was quick to tell me that she had not "cheated" on the recommendations I had given her previously about her diet. She had cut back on refined carbohydrates and had a new love for salmon. She also said that things in her life were pretty good and that her stress levels were under control. But when I asked her about changes in her skincare routine, that's where something struck me. Always game to try a new fad, Jennifer had started using trendy "extra gentle" facial exfoliators daily to "refresh and smooth" her skin. Because her skin was doing so well from our regimen, she thought these products would only enhance her healthy-looking skin, especially because they were touted as extra gentle. Not the case. All the rubbing from these scrubs was doing more harm than good. It was breaking down her skin's surface layer, allowing allergens and irritants to penetrate and stir up trouble. Her skin barrier was badly compromised, a situation that manifested itself as a severe rosacea flare-up.

Bowe Glow Tip

Even for my patients with supremely healthy skin, I recommend using a gentle scrub only twice per week at the most, and I advise entering these scrubbing days into your smartphone's calendar so you can keep diligent track of them and avoid overdoing it. It's such a common issue with my patients, and fixing it is very easy (and saves you money, too).

Jennifer's obsession with skin "cleansing" did not surprise me. Such a fixation is promoted everywhere. Flip on the TV during the day and you'll find plenty of commercials hawking the power of bleach and other chemicals to deep-clean and sanitize your house. You'll also see ads for products that de-germ your hands and remove 99.9 percent of viruses and bacteria "to help protect your family." With all this messaging about cleanliness and disinfecting, it's no wonder our minds are tainted when it comes to skin care. The cleaner your skin, the healthier it is, right? Wrong! We use harsh antibacterial soaps, alcohol-based toners, washcloths, loofahs, buff puffs, and body brushes in an effort to get that squeaky-clean feeling. Most dermatologists agree that the number one mistake people make when it comes to their skin-care regimen is overcleansing. In the short term, overcleansing will not be too disruptive, but chronically overcleansing—especially with strong cleansers—not only strips the skin of its natural oils but also wipes away those beneficial bacteria that actually keep your skin healthy!

As soon as Jennifer stopped the daily exfoliating scrubs, her skin began to heal. I also prescribed oral probiotics, live beneficial bacteria in pill form, to give her skin support from the inside out. Crisis averted. Within a month, Jennifer's skin was as vibrant and glowing as her personality, and we were back on track. As we'll see in detail in a later chapter, overwashing and overtreating the skin are among the most common culprits behind a bad complexion. Jennifer's experience reflects what countless other women go through when they mistake "cleanliness" for clear skin. Trying to get that super-pure feeling will only leave your skin angry and prone to a disorder. There is beauty in being "dirty."

Cassie, to cite another example, is one of the most fit, athletic women I know. She runs her own company, and exercise is her outlet — a productive way to clear her mind, focus her energy, and increase her productivity. In fact we often run into each other at a favorite fitness class that combines cardio and strength training. I admire her competitive spirit and her take-charge attitude.

I hadn't seen Cassie in a few months because she was traveling extensively for work. I did, however, notice that she was posting less frequently on social media about her exciting travels. I hoped everything was going well, because that was unusual for Cassie, who loves to share her adventures with friends and family back home.

When she returned, Cassie made an appointment and arrived in a panic. She had developed severe adult acne while she was away. She had never experienced acne as a teen, had never before dealt with it as an adult, and was not under any more stress than usual professionally or personally. She had stopped posting on social media because she was so self-conscious about her appearance. It had even started to affect her confidence at work.

We first talked about skin care: no noteworthy changes. Then we turned to her diet, which led to the culprit. As Cassie had become more devoted to her high-intensity workouts, she had also become hooked on a popular whey-based dietary supplement line that includes shakes, bars, and snacks—everything to help her build muscle and enhance her exercise regimen.

I had seen this exact combination—high-whey diets and adult acne—in several of my athletic patients. Recent scientific studies have established this link.[2] Unfortunately, the type of acne that arises from such high whey intake often cannot be resolved with typical acne treatments, including prescription topical and oral therapies. Given that Cassie didn't want to give up dietary supplements altogether, I encouraged her to try some plant-based options. No sooner did she make the change from whey to plant-based proteins than her acne began to resolve. Now I'm happy to say I see Cassie more at our exercise class than I do on my exam table, and she is looking and feeling fitter than ever before! At first glance, it may seem like Jennifer and Cassie have wildly different skin problems. But at their core, each reveals that the parts of the body are much more interconnected than we often imagine. And sometimes the solution to a skin problem is a holistic approach that has nothing to do with drugs.

Many of my patients are surprised when I ask them about what is generally going on in their lives, what they typically eat and drink, and how many times they use a facial exfoliant (if they do). They expect me to quickly prescribe medications, not knowing that this will merely mask their symptoms and leave the root of their problem untreated. Granted, sometimes prescriptions (oral and topical) are necessary and appropriate to help remedy a certain condition, as they were in Jennifer's case. But when my prescriptions don't work their magic as I expect them to, I know I have to dig deeper. That's when I have to look at a patient's diet, exercise, skin-care routine, and general lifestyle. To effectively address these issues, we must acknowledge one of the most remarkable discoveries of the modern era: the gut-brain-skin axis. Indeed, it is what all skin conditions have in common. And nurturing it provides the foundation for flawless skin, no matter what other treatments you use.

THE GUT-BRAIN-SKIN AXIS

I know what you're asking: To achieve flawless skin that everyone notices, what do you do? What should you eat, what should you avoid, and how should you treat your skin? To begin answering these questions, we must first answer another: What causes most skin problems today?

Answer: a weak or dysfunctioning gut-brain-skin axis. Simple as that. Your gut, your brain, and your skin share a profound relationship—they are all connected in powerful, surprising ways. Think of your gut and skin as links in a chain, with your brain clasping the links together. If there's a kink somewhere in the chain—an imbalance that disrupts this delicate interlinked axis—you will experience physical problems, from gut trouble to skin conditions. Once you bring this alliance into balance, beginning with your gut, you can see the results on the outside—and feel them on the inside. I'll be going into great detail about this axis in the next chapter, but for now here's a primer on the gut's connection to great skin.

YOUR GUT AS GROUND ZERO

The idea that the state of your gut dictates a lot about your health (and how you look) is not nearly as revolutionary as you might think, given its recent acceptance by modern medicine. Physicians from ancient Rome and Greece believed that illness often began in the colon. More than two thousand years ago, the Greek physician and father of modern Western medicine, Hippocrates, suggested that death sits in the gut (this is sometimes quoted as "All disease begins in the gut"). He also said, "Bad digestion is at the root of all evil"—a wise observation made long before civilization had any sound theory or scientific proof to explain it. In my practice, the patients with the most severe skin conditions often have gastrointestinal challenges as well.

Words to Warm Up To

Intestinal and skin flora: the symbiotic bacteria occurring naturally in the intestine and skin. A symbiotic relationship is one in which two species (e.g., bacteria and humans) live with each other in one of three ways: (a) both species benefit (mutualistic symbiosis), (b) one benefits and the other remains unharmed (commensal symbiosis), or (c) one benefits and the other is harmed (parasitic symbiosis).

Dysbiosis: a microbial imbalance on or inside the body (e.g., gut dysbiosis, skin dysbiosis).

Microbiome: the collection of microorganisms living in a particular environment, such as a human body or body part (e.g., the intestine, skin, mouth, nose, genitalia, or urinary tract). Microbiomes exist throughout nature, from the ocean floor and forests to other animals.

Microbiota: an ecological community of commensal, symbiotic, and pathogenic (potentially harmful) microorganisms found in and on all multicellular organisms.

We are walking ecosystems. You probably like to think of yourself as an individual, but when it comes to what lives in your body, you are far from alone. As you're beginning to appreciate (I hope!), you are home to trillions of invisible microbial organisms, mostly bacteria, that inhabit your insides and outsides. And your microbial comrades join you early in life. The current thinking is that while some microbes probably reach us in utero, the majority of the initial colonization happens when we descend through the birth canal and are exposed to organisms in the vagina. These microbes shower over us, causing our microbiomes to bloom at birth. The process continues as we begin life in the outside world. This may explain the difference between the lifetime health of babies born vaginally and the health of those born via a relatively sterile C-section. New science has revealed that C-section babies may not develop as diverse a microbiome and, as a result, can have a higher risk for certain conditions later in life—mostly inflammatory and immune problems (more on this later).[3]

We didn't know about these microbes just a few generations ago, but we have been evolving with them over millions of years. The two million unique bacterial genes found in each human microbiome can make our roughly twenty-three thousand or so genes pale by comparison. We are a "meta-organism," a living collective of microbes in and around us.[4] We need them for our survival. And we most definitely need them for beauty.

While it may make you uncomfortable to picture yourself completely covered inside and out with bacteria (both living and dead), as well as with fungi, yeasts, parasites, and viruses, it helps to remember that the friendly organisms are key to survival, and they do outnumber the villains in a healthy, balanced body. Good hygiene does not entail wiping out all germs. On the contrary, it involves cultivating, supporting, and maintaining beneficial bacteria and germs. In this way, you're optimizing your microbiome for health—both inside and out. And yes, that means getting dirty once in a while.

Your gut's microbial inhabitants, which are often collectively referred to as your intestinal flora, are workhorses.[5] They assist with digestion and the absorption of nutrients: you can't nourish yourself effectively without them. They also make and release important enzymes and other substances that your body requires but cannot generate in sufficient quantities on its own. These include vitamins (notably B vitamins) and neurotransmitters such as dopamine and serotonin. Get this: an estimated 90 percent of the feel-good hormone serotonin in your body is not made in your brain. It's produced in your digestive tract, thanks to your gut bugs. Your intestinal flora and their effects on your hormonal system help you handle stress and even get a good night's sleep. And your microbes participate in your metabolism. This means your microbes can influence your ability to maintain an ideal weight. It also means that your gut's microbes can affect your skin through the cascading effects of your metabolism (more on this shortly).

Of all the actions that these microscopic organisms perform to keep you healthy, perhaps the most vital are the ones that boost, regulate, and support your immune system—all of which is tied directly to the health of your skin.[6] Not only do intestinal microbes form a physical barrier against potential invaders (e.g., harmful viruses, parasites, and bad bacteria), they also act collectively as a giant detoxifier—they neutralize many toxins that reach your intestines via eating and drinking. They also help the immune system accurately distinguish between friend and foe and avoid dangerous allergic reactions and autoimmune responses. Some researchers assert that the alarming increase in autoimmune diseases in the Western world may be caused by a disruption in the body's long-standing relationship with its microbiome.[7]

Because gut bacteria can control certain immune cells and help manage the body's inflammatory pathways (see page 32), it is said that the gut (including its inhabitants) is akin to your immune system's largest "organ." Gut bacteria may ultimately affect your risk for all manner of chronic afflictions, from neuropsychiatric illnesses and degenerative brain disorders to autoimmune ailments, metabolic conditions such as obesity and diabetes, cancer, and, yes, dermatological issues—from acne to psoriasis, eczema, accelerated aging, and hair loss (in both males and females). And the common denominator here is inflammation, an important concept that I'll be reiterating throughout the book. Inflammation is key to survival, for it helps us recover from injury and fight infections. But when the inflammatory response is constantly "on" in the body, it can be an underlying cause of illness and disease.

The Ills of Inflammation

One of the most important discoveries in modern medicine has been the dangers of chronic inflammation. Inflammation is the process underlying every chronic illness and skin disorder. Even your mood is affected by bodily inflammation. Incidentally, there's also a stunning link between mood disorders and skin challenges.

Inflammation is two-faced: it has a good and a bad side. The good: inflammation helps you recover from illness or injury. As the body's natural healing mechanism, it temporarily amps up the immune system to take care of, say, a skinned knee or cold virus. But there's a downside to inflammation. When the process is always "on" and the immune system is permanently keyed up, the biological substances produced during the inflammatory process don't recede, and they begin to harm even healthy cells throughout the body. This type of inflammation is systemic—it's a slow-boil, full-body disturbance that is usually not confined to one particular area. The bloodstream allows it to spread to every part of the body. Fortunately we have the ability to detect this kind of widespread inflammation through blood tests.

Our bodies have a *symbiotic* relationship with our bacteria. A symbiont is an organism that lives together with another in a process called symbiosis. Symbiosis can be mutualistic, a relationship in which both organisms benefit; commensal, in which one organism benefits but the other is not harmed; or parasitic, in which one organism benefits and the other is harmed. The vast majority of human–microbiome interactions are mutualistic. Around the world, many microbiome research projects are under way, employing state-of-the-art technology to better understand how these bacterial symbionts influence our physiology. Not only are scientists documenting the microbial profiles of various microbiomes, they are also charged with figuring out which profiles relate to which conditions—for good or ill. No doubt this undertaking is monumental but momentous at the same time. And by some measures, these collective projects may become more significant and game-changing for medicine than the Human Genome Project.

Human microbiome research projects have already documented myriad functions of the microorganisms living in and on our bodies. As I stated, the gut can be considered the immune system's largest "organ," thanks to the presence and workings of its bugs. Well, it turns out that another reason for this is gut-associated lymphoid tissue (GALT), which surrounds the gut and is considered part of it. At least 80 percent of our body's total immune system is made up of GALT. Our immune system is headquartered in the gut because the intestinal wall is a biological gateway of sorts to the outside world, so aside from skin, it's where we have the greatest chance of encountering foreign material and organisms. The GALT communicates with other immune-system cells throughout the body, notifying them if cells in the gut encounter a potentially harmful substance. This is also why our food choices are so fundamental to immune health and, by implication, skin health: consuming the wrong things for you and your bugs could spell trouble from the perspective of the gut-based immune system. Conversely, eating the things that support, maintain, and enhance you and your bugs could be compared to having a platinum health insurance policy.

The skin, which is among the body's most important immune-related organs, has a parallel system called SALT: skin-associated lymphoid tissue. Your skin harbors trillions of lymphocytes that interact with the rest of the immune system via your lymph nodes. They also work in collaboration with the skin's microbial community. Unfortunately, we often think of skin as a surface that is relatively stable and needs to be clean. We fail to appreciate it as a complex organ that needs to be nurtured and protected. As I've witnessed in patients who don't properly take care of their skin and its microbiome, this can have a negative effect on skin health and even on the immune system over the long term.

THE SURPRISING RELATIONSHIPS BETWEEN GUT HEALTH, METABOLISM, AND SKIN HEALTH

Among the most revealing studies of the microbiome's influence on our health are those that show its impact on metabolism. Indeed, much of what we know about the intestinal microbiome has stemmed from studying its role in obesity and, conversely, its effect on our ability to stay lean. Bear with me, because when you understand the link between microbes and metabolism, you'll grasp the link between gut health and skin health. In fact the established science now shows that the microbial gut profiles of lean people resemble a dense, rich forest filled with many different species of bacteria. Those of obese people, on the other hand, are much less diverse. And, no, I've never met a patient who complained when my advice ended up clearing her skin *and* resulted in unexpected weight loss.

Evidence of gut bacteria affecting obesity and, by extension, metabolism has come from animal and human studies comparing intestinal bacteria in obese and lean subjects. The pioneering work of Drs. Jeffrey Gordon and Rob Knight have convincingly showed that the microbiome is closely linked with obesity. In their now famous 2013 sibling study, their team engineered baby mice to harbor microbes from either a lean or an obese woman.[8] These "humanized" mice were then put on the same diet in equal amounts. Then the researchers watched in awe as the mice that had the "fattening" microbial colonies grew heavier than the mice who were equipped with microbes from the lean woman. And the fat mice's gut microbes were much less diverse. The experiments continued in large enough numbers to prove that the condition of one's microbiome may be just as influential as, if not more influential than, both diet and genetics in controlling fat content! More research in humans is needed, but what the mouse models show thus far is enough to raise the flag.

What all this really means is that being overweight or obese is probably not necessarily a straightforward math problem of too many calories coming in and not enough calories getting burned. The latest research reveals that the microbiome likely plays a fundamental role in how much energy we use, which affects that calories in–calories out equation. If your gut contains too many microbial species that are adept at helping your body absorb calories from food, guess what: you'll extract more calories than you probably need from the foods you eat, leading to fat accumulation. The relationship between all this and your skin comes down to a common denominator: the gut's ecological health has a downstream impact on everything from your metabolism to your skin health.

I may be a dermatologist, but I love the fact that I can remedy so much more than skin problems for my patients. If you suffer from metabolic issues such as insulin resistance and diabetes, listen up: your gut microbiome's influence on your metabolism means it factors into blood-sugar balance and risk for metabolic dysfunction. An increasing amount of research being published in today's most prestigious medical journals is tracing the relationship between types of bugs in the gut and risk for insulin resistance and type 1 diabetes. I have my own anecdotal evidence, too, because many of my patients who follow my recommendations for their skin also find that their metabolic challenges lessen or — better yet — disappear! That's what is so exciting about this mission of mine now. It's incredibly rewarding.

As I'll be reiterating throughout the book, when you heal your gut, you heal so much more — and you'll see it when you look in the mirror. Later on, we'll explore how the health of your intestinal microbiome is affected not only by diet but also by hygiene (yes, dirty can be better than sanitized), levels of stress, exercise or lack thereof, and certain drugs, particularly antibiotics. There is now astonishing research showing the links between antibiotic use and obesity, as illustrated by the gut's microbial changes (as we'll see in chapter 5). The Gordon Lab, at Washington University, and the Knight Lab, at the University of California at San Diego, are among the leaders in the charge of helping us decode our microbiomes so we can understand how they make us who we are—and influence what we look like. Suffice it to say that your gut is among your body's most important keys to health and glowing skin.

YOUR SKIN HAS A MIND OF ITS OWN

Over the course of your lifetime, your body's largest organ serves as your interface with the world, around the clock, 365 days a year, and it works hard continuously. It doesn't take a vacation when you're on the beach soaking up the sun or outsource its job to any other organ. Given this, you can appreciate that it must be self-sufficient and well designed. It seems safe to say that no other organ of the body is exposed to such an expansive and diverse array of potential stressors as is the skin. It's bombarded by UV rays from the sun and by pollution, both of which create a steady stream of free radicals that act as missiles, targeting DNA, collagen, and even skin-cell membranes. The skin is exposed to allergens, irritants, and harmful pathogens that are constantly trying to get inside the body. Air pollution, in fact, is much more damaging to skin than previously thought. It may be invisible to the naked eye, but it can penetrate the skin and cause wrinkles and brown spots. Now more than ever we need to repair the skin barrier and keep skin's villains out.

In many ways, skin has a mind of its own. In fact the skin, brain, and central nervous system are much more closely tied together than you might think: they share the same tissue during development in utero. When you were nothing but a small embryonic bundle of cells, you were made up of two distinct layers: an ectoderm (outer layer) and an endoderm (inner layer). The outside layer, the ectodermal cells, was what became your nervous system as well as certain sensory organs, such as your eyes and ears, hair, nails, and teeth, the linings of your mouth, nose, and anal canal, and your skin and its glands. The inner layer, the endodermal cells, gave rise to the linings of your digestive tract, respiratory tract, bladder, and urethra. After these first two layers started to develop, a third layer, called the mesoderm (middle layer), began to grow, forming other interior elements such as blood, lymphoid tissue, bone, muscle, connective tissue, and the linings of other cavities.

Picturing your entire nervous system, including your brain, as being on the outside of your body is a little strange and counterintuitive, but that's where it is during a super-early stage of life, when an embryo has indistinguishable body parts. The brain, which isn't really a brain yet at that point, starts as an outer layer of cells and then eventually folds inward. Essentially this folding leaves your developing skin layer on the outside — a twin with a different job (and different types of cells in its makeup). I'd say that is quite an intimate relationship to share from the beginning.

One of the most fascinating scientific discoveries documented during my early days of training was that skin does not necessarily have to rely on the body's central stress-response system. It has its own built-in ability to respond to stress without getting "approval" or direction from the brain.[9] In fact it has established its own independent, parallel version of the famous hypothalamic-pituitary-adrenal (HPA) axis, which we'll explore in chapter 3. This "sister" system of the skin can even produce some of the same "fight or flight" chemicals, such as cortisol and endorphins, that are made and used by the body when it responds to stress. This means that when the skin is under attack — by environmental agents, harsh cleansers and soaps, the wrong diet, and even certain medications and cosmetics — cells in your skin spring into action and trigger a response that can result in a skin abnormality.

Let's back up a little. We have special organs that sit on top of our kidneys called adrenal glands. When our prehistoric ancestors encountered a menacing lion or bear, the adrenal glands triggered the release of adrenaline and another stress hormone called cortisol, which put their bodies into fight-or-flight mode so they could either run away fast or take on that ferocious beast. Now these hormones flood our system when we get called into the boss's office or feel overwhelmed. It's that same full-body response that helps give us an "adrenaline rush" to get us through a stressful time. Cortisol and adrenaline can make our hearts beat faster, our brains think quicker, and beads of sweat form on our brows.

Stress hormones are great to have when you encounter a serious threat or when you're gearing up to run a race or ace a test. They also serve an important role if you're fighting a serious infection or are going through major surgery. But these hormones, when released at low levels for long periods of time (for example, if you're not getting enough sleep or multitasking to an extreme), can actually be terribly detrimental to your overall health and the health of your skin.

As you can see, skin is pretty spectacular, even in comparison to its kindred spirit, the brain. The fact that skin can spark immune responses independently and produce some of the same substances we once thought were exclusive to the brain and nervous system is extraordinary. But this amazing capability also has its downsides, because those skin-directed responses can result in unwanted outcomes, such as acne, rosacea, psoriasis, and other troubling skin conditions. Your skin is your first line of defense against the danger-filled outer world, where you are susceptible to injury, stressors, and illness. It behooves us all to take care of our skin as we would any other vital organ.

The language that your skin and nervous system share is one that scientists are just beginning to translate. The area of medicine devoted to decoding and understanding this complex language is one of the hottest branches of skin research, right alongside the mapping of the skin's ecological biome—the mix of bacteria, yeasts, and parasites that live on it. As I've already mentioned, at any given time, trillions of organisms, including thousands of species of bacteria as well as viruses, fungi, and mites, live on your skin. Most of these microbes contribute to skin's function and health, though under certain circumstances the balance can be thrown out of whack and open you up to skin conditions.

STRENGTHENING OUR MICROBIAL ARMY

We're on the precipice of entering a "postantibiotic" era, thanks to the rise of antibiotic-resistant strains of bacteria.[10] Creating a paradigm shift in how we approach the skin, this rise is quickly becoming a serious game changer in my field and the entire skin-care industry. As a nation obsessed with that squeaky-clean feeling, we've been focused on wiping out bad bugs through antibiotics (topical and oral), antiseptics, and antibacterial soaps. But it has come at a steep cost. By overusing these items, we've started down the road to resistance, meaning that future generations might not be able to use these medicines at all—for anything. Imagine having a child diagnosed with a lifethreatening infection that was once easy to treat but for which there's no longer a remedy.

By some measures, antibiotics are needlessly prescribed or misused by patients in 50 percent of cases. When the wrong antibiotics are prescribed, or when they are prescribed unnecessarily, or when the person taking them uses them incorrectly (i.e., he or she doesn't take them for the full prescribed period or the medicine gets used sporadically rather than continuously—this happens a lot in my field), the door opens for harmful bacteria to mutate to the point where they no are longer affected by antibiotics. They become "immune" (resistant) to antibiotics, and we become unresponsive to these drugs. The creation of new strains of bad bacteria that are impervious to antibiotics paves the way for a dangerous situation wherein we no longer have drugs in our arsenal to combat the bacteria that cause harm and fuel abnormal skin conditions and systemic infections. I can't tell you how frequently I see patients who are on regimens of antibiotic acne medications that are no longer working because the acne harbors resistant strains of bacteria. The bacteria on their skin that contribute to their acne flares have become resistant to the antibiotics that once worked wonderfully. The bacteria themselves have changed in response to the antibiotic. And these resistant strains are difficult, if not impossible, to eradicate. They are like rogue villains who won't go away, making acne and a host of other ailments increasingly harder to treat.

Multidrug-resistant organisms are everywhere. Even our best pharmaceutical companies and researchers have not been able to develop new antibiotics despite extensive efforts during the first two decades of the twenty-first century. The situation is forcing us to take a gigantic pivot, but here's where there's good news: rather than wiping out the bad guys, we have started learning how to nurture and harness the good guys! We have to take advantage of the microbial army that lives in us and on our skin, defending us every day. In other words, we have to strengthen the *host,* not kill the enemy. Even major skin-care companies are recognizing that they have to test how their cleansers, creams, lotions, and even deodorants affect the microbiome. Are there certain ingredients that encourage the growth of healthy bacteria? Are there some ingredients that create a microbial environment that triggers inflammation? These are questions being addressed right now in skin-care R & D circles.

When we strengthen our microbial warriors, we empower them to help us fight enemies that can cause skin disorders as well as other ill-nesses and conditions. In the future, as scientific knowledge about our body's microbial world further develops, we will see an increasing number of probiotics and prebiotics hit the market to help us boost our microbiomes (both internally and externally). Whereas probiotics are live, active (friendly) cultures, prebiotics are fertilizerlike ingredients that promote the growth of beneficial microorganisms. To put it sim-ply, probiotics contain the good guys, and prebiotics contain what the good guys like to consume to ensure their own survival and prolifera-tion. Products like these can help nurture not only the good bacteria in our guts but also those that live on our skin and contribute to its health and functionality. I realize that some doctors today don't think much of probiotics, and they have doubts about whether they can in fact do anything when taken orally. In the past I have broken rank with my colleagues, and I will do so again on this topic because I truly believe we're on the cusp of an exciting new era in medicine (and dermatol-ogy) with respect to probiotics. Nowhere is the science of probiotics showing its powers more than in my field. We may not, for example, be able to cure conditions such as obesity easily and quickly with probiot-ics (yet), but there is a staggering amount of evidence that we'll soon have new solutions to skin challenges based in part on probiotic therapies.

One aspect of dermatological science that is really heating up and evolving has to do with understanding how topical probiotics that con-tain certain strains of bacteria can benefit our skin.[11] As we've come away from the antiquated idea that all bacteria are bad, we've come to realize that some kinds of bacteria can secrete natural antibiotics, improve hydration, support collagen production rather than collagen destruction, and produce other substances that are anti-inflammatory, soothing, and calming. Many beauty companies are investing heavily in research to identify which strains can address which skin problems as well as which strains can enhance overall appearance and skin health. I will be giving you guidance on how to find the best probiotic-infused skin-care products in addition to recipes for some simple DIY formulas you can make right at home in your kitchen.

Probiotics—both topical and ingested—can also offer protection from daily environmental stressors such as UV rays and pollution (both indoor and outdoor), which are the largest contributors to extrinsic aging. Ultraviolet light is not the only kind of light that can be damaging (any kind of light-induced damage to skin, by the way, is called photoaging). Infrared light has been shown to damage skin (watch out for hot yoga classes and saunas that use this wavelength to generate heat). New studies are even showing that visible light can create free radicals, damage the skin, and lead to discoloration in the skin (brown spots and patches that give you an uneven skin tone).[12] Visible light comes from computer screens, tablets, TVs, and from the typical indoor bulbs lighting your home and your office. However, the majority of scientists agree that the most threatening source of visible light and infrared light is the sun. Sunscreens on the market today, while effective against UV rays, are not effective at all against these other damaging rays. We'll discuss how to protect your skin against these assaults, both by using skin-care products and by making dietary changes. You'll never look at bell peppers, berries, dark chocolate, kimchi, yogurt, kombucha (say it with me: kom-BOO-cha), and dark leafy greens the same way again! (And yes, these are among the items you'll be adding to your grocery cart.)

THE BEAUTY MYTH

Your outer appearance is far from skin deep. One of the most widespread myths that I am constantly debunking is the notion that skin health is an isolated phenomenon—a surface problem. Much to the contrary, it's the upshot of myriad complex and highly regulated interactions that take place in the body, and it's affected by everything from your genome's behavior to that of the microbiome and its relationships with every system in your body, including your hormonal rhythms.

Another notion that circulates like a bad rumor is that flawless skin is genetic. You are not genetically destined to look like your mother or father. Yes, genes are part of the equation, but it's not as simple as all that. The DNA you were dealt is but one small slice of you. This means that there's a lot you can do to take control of your health and your looks. Although we are still just beginning to understand the human microbiome and how it relates to our physical health, including the appearance of our skin, evidence is quickly accumulating, giving us plenty of new "rules" on how to protect and support it as best we can. Even better, this book will lay out my three-week program to help you do just that.

In the future, I feel certain that we'll be able to identify microbial "profiles" of people who are prone to certain skin disorders and arrive at better preventive treatments. At the University of California at San Diego, an epicenter for cutting-edge research into the microbiome, Dr. Louis-Felix Nothias-Scaglia is biologically profiling the skin of people with psoriasis, which is a condition believed to be triggered by an overactive immune system. As Dr. Nothias-Scaglia explains, if molecules (metabolites) generated by certain bacteria are detected when the condition flares up, but not when the skin is psoriasis-free, we may be able to predict, by observing these microbial changes, when a psoriatic breakout is around the corner. And based on those molecules, we can figure out which drugs can treat the condition or prevent it altogether. This predictive knowledge would help patients expertly manage their psoriasis and reduce their use of potent immune-suppressing drugs that have unwanted side effects. Dr. Nothias-Scaglia works in the lab of Dr. Pieter Dorrestein, who uses mass spectrometry to "eaves-drop on the molecular conversations between microbes and their world."[13] By identifying our friendly microbes and their by-products, he hopes to gain a better picture of how microbes form communities and interact with one another and their environments (i.e., us). I envision a day when I can swab my patients' skin, have their microbiomes analyzed and profiled, and then custom-tailor a "prescription" to help them remedy a skin challenge or simply bring out their most beautiful, radiant selves. Microbiome sequencing will become routine in doctors' offices as we begin to build large databases that document and compare microbiomes based on age, skin type, and other demographic data. These databases will help inform how we doctors treat patients with skin conditions. It's initiatives like these that will allow us all to reap the rewards of truly personalized (precision) medicine.

Scientists are working to understand our microbiomes well enough to be able to manipulate them to achieve desirable outcomes. Imagine being able to tweak your gut microbial profile to help you effortlessly lose weight, terminate type 2 diabetes, reduce your risk for depression, dementia, and cancer, and support skin health. Similarly, imagine shifting the skin's microbial characteristics to thwart acne outbreaks, block UV rays and prevent skin cancer, deflect mosquitoes (indeed, new research shows that the microbes on our skin affect whether or not we are bitten), and usher in that coveted healthy glow. That's the promise that this exciting field of medicine has to offer. Time to get ready for it.

KNOW BEFORE YOU GLOW: THE SELF-CHECK

Consumer microbial kits that allow you to collect samples from your skin (or stool or mouth) and send it off to a company for profiling are beginning to emerge. But these tests—and the scientific data behind their results—need more time to incubate in the halls of research before they can tell us anything truly helpful on an individual basis. There is no foolproof test available today that can accurately tell you exactly the state of your microbiome, but you *can* gather some valuable clues by answering a few simple questions. This will also help you understand which experiences in your life may have affected the health of your microbiome—both during your youth and afterward. I've put the following self-assessment together for you to use.

Don't be alarmed if you find yourself answering yes to most of these questions. They are intended to assess your risk for dysfunctional physiology that might be affecting your health in general and your skin's health and function in particular—and demystifying the issues at hand is the first step to solving them.

You might wonder how some of these questions relate to skin health, but you'll soon have a full understanding from the lessons in this book. And if any particular question triggers you to ask further questions, rest assured that I will answer them in the following chapters. For now, just respond to these questions to the best of your ability and make note of which ones you answer in the affirmative.

What Are Your Risk Factors?

The quiz below will arm you with some personal data that can help provide a sense of your overall health and your risk factors for skin disorders and accelerated aging. Respond as truthfully as possible, but if you don't know the answer to a question, skip it.

1. Do you suffer from any skin conditions?
2. Do you have thinning hair, thinning brows or lashes, and/or brittle nails that aren't the result of a medically diagnosed nondermatological condition? (Many women don't think their hair is thin, but

they do notice that they are finding more hairs than usual in their brushes or shower drains.)

3. Do you suffer from chronic gastrointestinal issues such as constipation or diarrhea, gas, bloating, abdominal cramping or discomfort, IBS, bad breath, or acid reflux?

4. Have you ever been diagnosed with an autoimmune disorder (e.g., psoriasis, lupus, inflammatory bowel disease, rheumatoid arthritis)?

5. Do you feel like your skin is aging faster than it should?

6. Are you more than twenty pounds overweight?

7. Have you been diagnosed with type 2 diabetes or high blood sugar?

8. Have you taken antibiotics or used them on your skin at least once in the past two years?

9. Do you consume artificial sweeteners (e.g., Equal, Splenda) and low-calorie "diet" foods or beverages that are labeled and marketed as such?

10. Do you eat a lot of processed packaged convenience foods?

11. Do you experience insomnia or chronic sleep deprivation?

12. Do you avoid exercise?

13. Do you feel stressed out and overwhelmed most days of the week?

14. Are you extra sensitive to ingredients found in cosmetics, skin-care preparations, and beauty products?

15. Do you live in an urban environment?

16. Do you like to use saunas, spend time in steam rooms, or do hot yoga?

17. Have you ever had a bad sunburn or used tanning salons?

18. Were you born by C-section?

19. Do you use hand sanitizers or antibacterial soaps regularly?

20. Do you drink skim milk or protein shakes made with whey?

If you answered yes to five or more questions, then your skin is suffering needlessly and can benefit tremendously from the information in this book. Even if you only answered yes to one or two questions, you can help change the look and feel of your skin for the better. Curious as to how these questions (and their answers) relate to your skin? Read on to learn everything you want—and need—to know for a brighter and better-looking you.

Online Resources

Don't forget to go to my website, at www.DrWhitneyBowe.com, for scientific updates and my personal recommendations. This field is changing swiftly. I will keep up with it all and use my site as a repository of curated information and resources.

CHAPTER 2

The New Science of Skin

Understanding the Gut-Brain-Skin Connection

Andrea was like many of the women I meet in my office: beauty-conscious and struggling with stubborn skin issues for which she'd tried lots of do-it-yourself solutions she'd read about online. At thirty-five years old, she was suffering from persistent breakouts, blotchiness and redness, and an uneven skin tone. Products she was using in an attempt to relieve her problems stung her face and caused it to flake. She thought she was doing everything right: eating organic low-fat foods, using an expensive "purifying" cleanser with botanical enzymes on her face twice a day, and doing juice cleanses over the weekends to, in her words, "wipe out the toxins" that were ruining her complexion. Her juice cleanses were also an attempt to lose weight, for Andrea was hoping to drop the thirty pounds she'd gained since she was in her twenties. She couldn't understand what she was doing wrong until I began asking her questions that probed deeply into her nutritional and skin-care habits.

Contrary to Andrea's belief that she was eating healthfully, her diet was sabotaging her skin's ability to heal itself. On most days, she ate an organic energy bar or drank a protein shake made with skim milk for breakfast, picked up an iced caffè mocha next to her office midmorning, and switched to Diet Coke in the afternoon. For lunch she'd typically eat a salad with low-fat dressing or a sandwich with fat-free mayonnaise. She kept low-calorie rice cakes and pretzels on hand for snacking. I gave her credit for working out regularly (Andrea loved her SoulCycle classes and boot-camp workouts), but she lost points for imbalances in her exercise regimen. Like many of my patients, Andrea worked out seven days a week, focusing on high-intensity cardio but shunning exercises that address flexibility and strength. I also sensed that she led a super-busy work life as a lawyer in a big firm and was always on the go, so stress had to be a factor, too. Her body—and skin—were burned out.

"Your skin is inflamed because your gut is inflamed," I said to her. "In fact your whole body is probably on fire. And the way you treat your skin in the morning and at night is exacerbating everything."

I then went on to tell her about the connection between gut health and skin health and the value of being *dirty,* so to speak. I confiscated the hand sanitizer that she had in her purse, gave her new dietary and fitness guidelines, and put her on a new skin-care program tailored to nurture her skin's microbiome. As you know by now, our skin houses microbial colonies that are as much a part of our skin's health and functionality as our actual skin cells. When Andrea (or anyone else) routinely washes her face with caustic cleansers and abrasive buffs, she effectively kills off the good bacteria needed to foster radiant, clear skin. She also runs the risk of compromising her skin's natural barrier. The combination of her new skin-care routine, which consists of a gentle daily cleanser and the *occasional* use of an exfoliant, plus her dietary swaps (see page 208) and a more balanced approach toward exercise (exchanging two days of high-intensity cardio for yoga or Pilates), helped Andrea put out the flames that were igniting her skin condition.

Within two weeks, she saw results—results that reflected both a healthier gut-brain-skin axis and a better-balanced microbiome on her skin. Her skin tone brightened, the blotchy redness faded, and her breakouts subsided significantly. She dropped five pounds, too. Plus she felt fantastic. From there we went to work on helping her reduce her overall stress levels, which I knew had been contributing to her body's chaos and angry skin. I encouraged her to take more time for herself in the form of mindful walks in nature or thirty minutes to an hour over the weekend doing something calming, such as reading for pleasure, getting a pedicure, or talking to a friend.

THE DIRTY TRUTH

Andrea's experience is not an anomaly. As I've mentioned, every day I treat a wide variety of patients whose health issues manifest themselves in skin disorders but whose core troubles reside primarily in the gut— in those delicate folds of the intestines, where colonies of microbes thrive and influence our physiology. Indeed, the body's microbiome exerts an enormous force on our biology—so much so that it's believed it may affect our health as much as or more than the genes we inherit from our parents. And while Andrea thought she was "doomed to be fat" because her parents were both overweight, I explained to her that new scientific evidence is showing that the body's community of friendly germs has the power to affect its metabolism and even speak to its own genome, changing how it behaves. The bacteria, whose genetic information eclipses our own DNA in volume, can turn our genes on or off. These bacteria are one of the body's remote controls: they help determine such things as whether we gain or lose weight and whether we have amazing or awful skin. No one is necessarily "doomed" by his or her inherited genes. Far from it.

HISTORY REPEATS ITSELF

Surprisingly, the discovery of the link between gut health and skin health is not a twenty-first-century "Eureka!" event. Researchers as far back as 1930 suspected a connection, but our modern scientific tools have allowed us to finally confirm the importance of this relationship. It hinges on the balance of bacteria in our intestines as well as on the condition of the intestinal wall.

At Andrea's first appointment with me, my mind immediately went to the state of her microbiome. My educated guess was that it was sick, overrun with unfriendly bacteria. Her intestinal wall was probably "leaky," too. One of the key issues that intestinal bacteria help control is your gut's permeability. If a microbial disturbance causes problems with the integrity of the cells lining the gut, it will affect the passage of nutrients from the digestive tube into the body. A leaky intestinal wall will fail to appropriately police what should be allowed in (nutrients) and kept out (pathogens that trigger an immune response and inflammation).

The concept of a "leaky gut" was once viewed as a dubious theory by conventional researchers and doctors, but now an impressive number of well-designed studies have repeatedly shown that when your intestinal barrier is damaged, it can result in the proliferation of unhealthy gut flora unable to protect the integrity of the intestinal lining. This leaves you susceptible to a whole spectrum of health challenges, skin disorders chief among them. You can also have "leaky skin," a condition in which the skin's natural barrier is broken. As you can imagine, skin's chief role is to act as a fence—it is what stands between us and the outside world. While it protects us from many different types of external threats, such as harmful substances, UV rays, and pathogens, it also helps prevent the escape of the precious water in our bodies. If this barrier is compromised somehow, harmful substances can pass through the skin's layers. In people who have rosacea and eczema, for example, an impaired skin barrier leads to a loss of hydration (skin can't trap moisture); this combination of factors enables allergens and irritants from the environment to deeply penetrate the outer layer and trigger inflammation. Research demonstrates that the skin's barrier is also damaged by stress—both psychological and physical (what one scientist calls "a nervous breakdown in the skin").[1] So whether you are struggling with an illness, enduring a painful divorce, or recovering from surgery, your body registers that as stress, which will affect your brain, your gut, and, in turn, your skin.

SKIN GETS STRESSED OUT

In 2011, I cowrote one of the first academic papers to bring the gut-brain-skin axis into the spotlight, especially as it relates to acne.[2] But our understanding of the gut-brain-skin axis began in 1930, in a study that looked at the effects of one particular type of stress on the body: psychological, or emotional, stress. Two revered American dermatologists, John H. Stokes and Donald M. Pillsbury, based at the University of Pennsylvania, first proposed a gastrointestinal explanation for the relationship between the state of one's skin and psychological conditions such as depression and anxiety.[3] At the time, in the medical field, there was a growing interest in studying and documenting the effects of emotions and nervous states on bodily function. When these prescient doctors set out to look at such effects on skin health, their specialty, they hypothesized that emotional states might change the normal gut flora, increase intestinal permeability (triggering leaky gut), and contribute to widespread inflammation—which, as you know, extends to the skin. Some of the remedies they suggested were *Lactobacillus acidophilus* cultures—a common probiotic found in many cultured yogurts and other fermented foods.

The bond between the mind and skin has long-established roots. Skin-to-skin contact between a newborn and its mother surely is part of those roots. Recall that the brain and skin grow from the same embryonic layer in a developing fetus. That alone says a lot about the ingrained bond between these two seemingly disparate organs and systems. In fact it is this very bond that gives us one of our most basic interfaces with the world: our sense of touch. It's really no surprise that our emotions affect our skin—they have a relationship that is equal parts intimate and intricate.

Since Stokes and Pillsbury's work, the association between chronic skin conditions and mental health disorders has been recognized in medical literature, particularly the idea that intestinal microflora, inflammatory skin conditions, and psychological symptoms such as depression are all physiologically intertwined. But only since the late 1990s or so has there been a focus on interpreting the interaction between the brain (and nervous system in general) and skin diseases. Psychodermatology, or psychocutaneous medicine, is a new subspecialty in medicine that's emerging from the combination of psychiatry and dermatology.[4] Whereas in psychiatry one studies and treats mental processes manifested internally, in dermatology one generally studies and treats skin diseases manifested externally. (Keep in mind it can be a bit of a self-fulfilling prophecy: having skin conditions can fuel anxiety and depression because of disfiguring or unpleasant effects that change or diminish one's appearance.)

All of us have "felt" the gut-brain-skin connection: think of the last time you were under acute stress, were exceptionally nervous, scared, or anxious, or felt deeply embarrassed. Maybe it was before meeting a potential new employer, after tripping in front of a crowd, or while walking down the aisle at your wedding. Suddenly you felt sick to your stomach or, in the case of feeling humiliated, you blushed. Consider a time when you've gotten goose bumps or felt your skin crawl, or when you experienced the sudden sensation of feeling hot and sweaty because you were about to face your fear of heights by zooming across a zip line. That is the least scientific — but most relatable — evidence I can provide to explain the link between the gut and brain (and skin!). These powerful links work in multiple directions. Just as your brain can send butterflies to your stomach and blood to your face, causing you to blush, your gut can relay its state of alarm or calm to your nervous system and ultimately change your skin's appearance. Allow me to explain some of the hardwiring that's going on here.

Your nervous system comprises more than your brain and spinal cord. In addition to this central nervous system, you have an intestinal, or *enteric*, nervous system that is part of the gastrointestinal tract. As previously mentioned, these two systems are created from the same tissue during fetal development. The vagus nerve, which extends from the brain stem to the abdomen, is the primary channel of information between the millions of nerve cells — anywhere from two hundred million to six hundred million — in your central and enteric nervous systems. The vagus nerve is the longest of the twelve pairs of cranial nerves and is sometimes referred to as cranial nerve X, because it is numbered as the tenth in the lineup of nerve pairs in the brain. It also forms part of the nervous system that controls many bodily processes that don't require conscious thinking, such as digestion and heart rate.

Because the enteric nervous system depends on the same types of neurons and neurotransmitters that are found in the brain and spinal cord (central nervous system), it is fondly referred to as a "second brain." When neurons lining the digestive tract sense that food has entered the gut, these neurons signal muscle cells to commence a series of intestinal contractions that move food farther along. As the food moves down, it gets broken into either nutrients for absorption or waste for removal. The enteric nervous system also uses neurotransmitters such as serotonin (made by the gut bugs) to communicate and interact with your body's central nervous system.[5]

For many of my patients, the importance of gaining control of stress as a path to achieving better skin health means eating better, establishing the right skin-care routine, and taking the proper medications for their conditions. In fact I sometimes wonder if managing stress successfully has as much of an effect on skin health as good dietary habits. The mind and the skin are intimately intertwined, which we'll explore in even more depth in chapter 3. This topic is deserving of its own chapter: my goal here is only to give you a primer and general overview of the gut-brain-skin axis—especially as it relates to psychology.

Many skin disorders—acne, rosacea, eczema, psoriasis, alopecia (hair loss), and discoloration—take their roots from or place their roots in the psyche. When you maintain a calm mind, you can maintain calm skin. Generally speaking, sudden anxiety ("I just got pulled over for speeding!") or being temporarily nervous ("I don't think I'll make it through this speech!") can be a nuisance, but it's not particularly damaging to the microbiome or skin. Destructive stress, on the other hand, is the unabating kind, which can have more serious effects on the gut and skin. To understand these effects, it helps to know about SIBO: small intestinal bacterial overgrowth.

SIBO ON THE INSIDE, BAD SKIN ON THE OUTSIDE

Prolonged stress, which millions of people shoulder daily while keeping up with work, family, household responsibilities, and current events, does a number on the small intestine. Studies show that prolonged stress stagnates digestion in the intestine, which leads to an overgrowth of bacteria that then compromises the intestinal barrier (see page 58). This unfortunate series of events is often worsened by the typical Western diet, heavy in processed foods and low in fiber.

Fiber keeps the digestive system running like a well-oiled machine, but it's important for other reasons. Fiber is what fuels the growth of good bacteria in the gut. In the absence of plentiful fiber, digestion slows and unfriendly bacteria are allowed to grow, crowding out the beneficial bugs and changing the gut composition. This then leads to a host of negative effects, from digestive disorders to skin disorders. So it's a double whammy when you're stressed out *and* eating a low-fiber diet: SIBO is highly likely. SIBO also results when certain bacteria from the colon inhabit the small intestine, where they don't belong.

First documented by Stokes and Pillsbury, SIBO can manifest itself in a variety of ways, ranging from a lack of noticeable symptoms to severe malabsorption syndrome, which makes it difficult to properly absorb needed proteins, carbohydrates, fats, vitamins, and minerals. It often manifests itself as gastrointestinal symptoms, including bloating, abdominal pain, diarrhea, bad breath, acid reflux, and sometimes constipation. SIBO is also known to be prevalent in people suffering from anxiety and depression as well as those diagnosed with ailments such as fibromyalgia and chronic fatigue syndrome—conditions characterized by an impairment of the normal function of a bodily process without a visible physical abnormality.★

The excess bad bacteria at the root of severe malabsorption can compete with the body for nutrients, produce toxic by-products, and cause direct injury to cells in the small intestine. The resulting

---

★ Clinical tests are available today to try and diagnose SIBO. These tests, most of which are breath tests performed over several hours, do have their limitations and won't tell you the root cause of the problem. If you have classic symptoms of SIBO, such as chronic gas, bloating, abdominal pain/ cramps, and diarrhea, you may want to consider seeing a gastroenterologist for treatment in addition to using the program in this book. Note that SIBO can have overlapping symptoms with many other gastrointestinal disorders, particularly IBS.

inflammation-run-amok directly affects the skin. How so? Well, as the bad gut bugs outnumber the good gut bugs, the lining of the gut can become compromised. What's more, this microbial disruption increases susceptibility to intestinal pathogens and infection. A leaky gut then allows toxins to enter the bloodstream that would otherwise stay in the intestines and be properly neutralized or excreted. The combination of changes to the functionality of the gut and the gut's microbiome spells trouble — trouble that can reach the skin. As the gut's overall integrity is compromised, the stage is set for widespread inflammation that is both systemic and local to the skin. Any systemic inflammation can manifest itself in skin conditions (among other health challenges). Which skin condition results depends on one's underlying vulnerabilities and genetics. You may be prone to acne or rosacea, whereas someone else may be prone to psoriasis or eczema.

On the next page is an illustration of SIBO from the paper I copublished in 2011 with Alan C. Logan of Canada's Royal Sociey of Public Health. It offers a visual summary of what I've just described.

The point is, the combination of a nutrient-poor diet and high stress levels sets one up for any number of skin challenges, which is why the program in this book offers methods to manage stress, a list of foods and ingredients to avoid, and a multitude of ideas for replenishing and nourishing a healthy gut, including suggestions for harnessing the power of probiotics. New studies are showing that probiotics — again, orally administered good bacteria, or live cultures — can have a profound impact on the gut's microbial community and on how it behaves.[6] Probiotics aside, I should point out that dietary change alone can be powerful. High-profile studies in which subjects did not take probiotics but improved their gut health simply by eating diets low in processed foods and sugars reported improvements in the subjects' skin, including a decrease in pus bumps and blackheads.[7] So the combination of probiotics and dietary change is like a one-two punch against skin

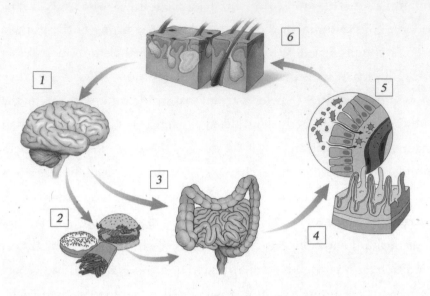

(1) Psychological distress, alone or in combination with (2) processed foods devoid of fiber, ends up slowing digestion. This in turn changes the type and number of bacteria that live in the gut and gut lining (3). This has been shown to lead to (4) increased intestinal permeability ("leaky gut"); the gut lining can become compromised, and toxins that are supposed to stay housed in the gut are released into the bloodstream (5), causing inflammation throughout the body, including in the skin (6). In people susceptible to acne, for example, this cascade is thought to influence the skin and potentially exacerbate the condition. Other people might be vulnerable to rosacea or psoriasis as a result of this cascade.
Printed with permission. © *Marcia Harstock, MA CMI*

disorders. Add stress-reducing strategies and you've got yourself a solution.

I rarely see a patient suffering from a chronic skin disorder who does not also suffer from an imbalance elsewhere in the body. Most of my patients complain of the same gastrointestinal issues that Pillsbury and Stokes wrote about in 1930—issues that further heighten their stress levels. A 2008 study, published in the *Journal of Dermatology,* involving more than thirteen thousand adolescents in China showed that those with acne were likely to experience gastrointestinal symptoms such as constipation, bad breath, and gastric reflux.[8] More specifically, abdominal bloating was 37 percent more likely to be associated with acne and other diseases related to oil-secreting glands. Some of the worst cases of acne I've seen are in patients who also have inflammatory bowel disease (ulcerative colitis, or Crohn's disease), which likely owes some of its origins to a disrupted microbiome. This is really no surprise, given the accumulating evidence about the power of the intestinal microbiome and its relation to the rest of the body. Andrea, whom I introduced at the start of this chapter, herself admitted to having frequent bloating and chronic heartburn, for which she self-medicated with Prilosec. These were more clues that her gut's microbial community was imbalanced and further inflaming her skin.

One major dietary culprit in cases of bad skin that surprises my patients when I mention it, as I did with Andrea, is diet soft drinks. Too many of us are under the impression that they are somehow better for us than soft drinks made with real sugar. Well, get this: studies of the effects of artificial sweeteners on the microbiome are downright jaw-dropping (I had to put down my diet iced tea immediately!).[9] The Splendas and Equals of the world may not contain calories, but they contain chemicals that have the power to disrupt the gut's microbial inhabitants so much that they negatively affect metabolism and blood-sugar balance. Those diet foods and beverages not only increase the risk of insulin resistance and diabetes, they also increase the risk of skin disorders such as acne and rosacea through the domino effect of increased inflammation. There are some sugar-substitute exceptions, however, that you can use in moderation that will be listed in chapter 10. Stevia (extracted from the leaves of a plant) and sugar alcohols such as xylitol are allowable. These sweeteners do not have the same impact on the body as classic artificial sugars do..

Another common ingredient has also gone down in the flames of good research. In 2015, laboratory studies revealed the injurious ramifications of dietary emulsifiers on the microbiome.[10] Just what are these gut — and skin — villains? Emulsifiers are molecules that act as blending agents in food products that contain otherwise unmixable ingredients, such as oil and water. They also act as preservatives. (I'm referring to emulsifiers that are added to foods — not naturally occurring emulsifiers in nutritious foods such as egg yolks and mustard.) Don't think you eat these food additives? They're in all manner of commercially processed foods, including ice cream, salad dressing, and cream cheese. You won't see the word *emulsifier* on the label, though. They are called by other unfamiliar names: carrageenan, soy lecithin, polysorbate 80, polyglycerols, guar gum, locust bean gum, and xanthan gum. Many of my patients' diets are filled with these gut disrupters that factor into their skin's appearance (until I set them straight on a new diet). When consumed, these substances adversely change the composition of the gut's microbiome, which in turn results in greater systemic inflammation, which can cause skin disorders.

GUT REBOOT TO GORGEOUS SKIN

I've said it once, and I'll say it again: diet is the most critical factor in the quest for gorgeous skin. Processed foods that lack fiber and are filled with low-quality artificial ingredients and additives are the number one offenders, resulting in a disrupted gut ecology that manifests itself in skin problems (among other ailments). And when you add psychological stress to poor diet, the impact on skin can be even more detrimental. This downward spiral is exactly what Andrea was experiencing. In addition to her general high stress levels, her diet was dominated by microbe-busting, pro-inflammatory foods that lacked the fiber contained in whole foods and the anti-inflammatory omega–3 fats in fish, olive oil, nuts, and seeds (she was from the generation that believed fat made you fat, so she tried to avoid it at all costs).

Andrea was well on her way to glowing, clear skin once we rebooted her gut through her diet. One important question she asked me once she began to see results was this: "I feel like I'm eating more now, but I'm losing weight practically effortlessly *and* my skin is clearing up. How is this possible?!"

I assured her that her body's microbiome was finally in sync with the rest of her body. She was burning calories more efficiently, absorbing more healthful nutrients, and controlling systemwide levels of inflammation. And her great skin was reflecting the harmony.

You'll soon be achieving the same goal: establishing a microbiome that works *with* you, not against you. So even though you may feel you're fighting an uphill battle, you have the potential to cultivate a balanced, healthy ecosystem within. We all do!

Andrea's Dietary Edits

The goal: remove pro-inflammatory, gut-unfriendly foods and introduce anti-inflammatory, gut-friendly choices that rehabilitate the body's beneficial flora. Studies show that gut flora can begin to change *within three days* and that lasting, long-term results in the skin can be measured within two weeks.

NO ➡ YES

Skim milk ➡ Organic, unsweetened coconut milk or almond milk

Low-fat and nonfat foods ➡ Healthful fats from fish, nuts, flaxseed, avocados, olive oil

Artificial sweeteners ➡ Real sugar and natural sugar substitutes in moderation

Juices from fruits ➡ Juices from greens (e.g., spinach, kale)

Caffè mocha ➠ Cappuccino or latte with unsweetened almond milk

Diet iced tea ➠ Homemade iced green tea

Whey protein powder ➠ Plant-based protein powder

High-glycemic foods* (sugary cereals, white rice, bagels) ➠ Low-glycemic foods (plain Greek-style yogurt, legumes, nonstarchy vegetables)

*I'll cover the importance of low-glycemic foods in chapter 6. These are foods that won't raise blood sugar significantly. Unfortunately, high-glycemic foods are ubiquitous today. They are not just found in processed, packaged foods (including the low-calorie rice cakes and pretzels Andrea loved) but also in seemingly innocuous fare such as melons, couscous, rice, raisins, and fava beans.

In this chapter, you've begun to get a sense of the gut–brain–skin axis and how your emotions and psyche (i.e., psychological stress) can influence the body and skin. But the relationship between your state of mind and your appearance is even more complex than I've described thus far. Only since the late 1990s have we been discovering how the body's nervous system, immune system, hormonal system, and skin communicate with each other. This extraordinary network ties directly into the microbiome. Let's go there next.

CHAPTER 3

Mind over Skin Matters

The Brain's Influence on the Body, Inside and Out

Patients often say to me: "Dr. Bowe, I feel like I aged ten years overnight!" Early on in my practice, I was skeptical of these dramatic statements and just assumed that my patients had started paying closer attention now that their fortieth or fiftieth birthdays were approaching, or maybe they just saw unflattering photos of themselves on social media. But as I became a more experienced dermatologist and started following my patients over time, I actually *witnessed* it happening—a forty-year-old patient whom I had been treating for a skin condition that required monthly visits all of a sudden appeared to age ten years in a short time period. Alison had developed fine lines around her eyes and mouth and brown spots on her chest, and her skin looked dry and dull and felt rough to the touch. She confided in me that her mother had fallen ill, and she was trying to care for her as well as raise three young children at home. The stress had taken its toll, and her skin was showing the signs.

The mind indeed wields a lot of power over the body and one's looks. But how, exactly? What's the underlying biology of this phenomenon? How can what you think—what your mental state is— translate to real, noticeable, tangible matters of skin health?

For a long time we physicians had a hard time understanding—and explaining—the connection between psychological health and physical health. Or how feeling under uncomfortable pressure for a prolonged period of time can trigger a wide range of bona fide conditions and illnesses. Dermatologists have long known that psychological stress often makes a patient's symptoms worse. If she has acne, psoriasis, eczema, or rosacea—any of the Big Four—these conditions are amplified during periods of high stress. Is it really coincidence that you break out during finals week, before your wedding, or after the death of a loved one? (And yes, stress takes many forms, including deeply felt emotions such as grief, shock, sadness, and profound disappointment.)

Today we know a lot more about the relationship between stress and health than ever before. In this chapter, I'll detail the specifics about the biology behind this relationship, focusing mostly on its impact on skin. Many skin and hair conditions—eczema, acne, psoriasis, alopecia— are greatly exacerbated by stress.

As you've learned by now, stress and anxiety affect the microbiome. And SIBO (small intestinal bacterial overgrowth) is one of the factors making it a two-way street: while gut bacteria can influence the brain and skin, signals can go *the other way*—especially from the brain to the gut. In the presence of psychological stress, this often manifests itself as both gastrointestinal and skin issues. As I mentioned, in my practice I frequently see patients with skin issues (e.g., acne, inflamed skin, premature aging, bags and papery skin around their eyes, broken blood vessels) who further struggle with GI problems as well as with anxiety and insomnia. I've come to learn that if a skin condition doesn't respond to my first line of therapy, it usually means I need to go further and identify an underlying source of stress. There's almost always a difficult, sometimes traumatic situation my patient is dealing with that's causing her to fight an uphill battle when trying to resolve a skin condition. Sometimes I do feel like my role as a doctor includes serving as a confidante whenever my patients visit. I listen with an open heart to their stories and learn about their family dynamics, deepest vulnerabilities, and insecurities. I keep their secrets sacred and do what I can to help them heal inside and out.

Looks Don't Lie

Another way to see the brain-skin link in action is to look at people in high-stakes, demanding jobs who are constantly under scrutiny by the public—elected heads of state, for example. Comparing photos taken before they were in office with photos taken after they've been in office a while can be revealing. Notice the graying, thinning hair; the lines, folds, and wrinkles in the skin; and the dark under-eye circles. These changes appear relatively quickly on them in comparison to their peers. The changes are not merely the effects of chronological aging. They are also the long-term effects of prolonged stress and anxiety on skin, hair, and nails. Bottom line: ongoing, unremitting stress triggers chronic inflammation that can lead to myriad skin issues.

STRESS AGING

Stress is an interesting word and concept. It has both a biological and sociological meaning. Broadly speaking, the word *stress* can refer to any real or perceived threat to the balance (homeostasis) of an organism. Stress, which can come from our lifestyle or the environment, can be sudden and temporary (acute) or pervasive and ongoing (chronic), the latter of which, as you know, tends to be the most damaging to health.

Most of us can recognize stress when we're experiencing it. If you had to articulate the feeling of stress, you'd probably say something about being irritated, anxious, maybe even sad. There can be a sense of impending doom—*something bad will happen.* Your heart might race and your face might redden if it's really acute stress, and you may experience more serious symptoms such as an upset stomach or a massive headache. Perhaps a big zit will start to develop on your face or you'll have a more widespread breakout. Everyone weathers stress differently. For some people, stress has little visible effect. Rather, it is internalized and can be detected by measuring blood pressure, stress hormones, and levels of inflammation. Sometimes it's detected by the onset of a chronic disease.

Generally speaking, we experience stress when the demands placed on us challenge our ability to cope. Our feelings, thoughts, and behaviors as well as the physiological changes that result from our response to those demands are also part of stress. Stress physiology has been studied a lot since the early twentieth century, and the field has gained considerable traction since the mid-twentieth century, thanks to major advances in medicine.

Stressors Old and New: Signs of the Times

Our great-grandparents had very different stressors from the ones that afflict us today. For example, they had to worry about infectious communicable diseases that could kill them quickly, whereas we're more likely to succumb to diseases slowly, over time, as we develop noncommunicable age-related ailments—heart disease, cerebrovascular illness, dementia, and many types of cancer. These conditions tend to build up subtly over many decades and present themselves either when we are vulnerable physically or when we're simply enfeebled by age.

In 1936, in the first scientific publication on the subject, one of the founding fathers of stress research, Hans Selye, defined biologic stress (what he called "general adaptation syndrome") as "the non-specific response of the body to any demand for change."[1] His work came on the heels of that of his predecessor Dr. Walter Bradford Cannon, who was chairman of the department of physiology at Harvard Medical School and coined the term *fight or flight* to describe an animal's response to threats.[2] Selye proposed that when subjected to persistent stress, both humans and animals could develop certain life-threatening afflictions, such as heart attacks and strokes, that previously were thought to be caused only by specific pathogens. This was a crucial revelation because it pointed to the impact that everyday life and experiences have on our physical health. Cannon was just twenty-six years old when his paper was published in the journal *Nature*.

There are an untold number of ways in which our thoughts and feelings both reflect and influence what goes on inside our bodies. And we now have an impressive body of scientific research to explain the complex intertwining of our psychology and overall biology. Intangibles such as emotional states (distress versus contentment), thought processes (the glass is half full versus half empty), and even socioeconomic status (rich versus poor) can all modify bodily functions and affect our digestion, metabolism, immunity, nerves, hormones, quality of sleep, and even skin cells. The paradox, of course, is that stress isn't always a crook trying to steal our health and beauty. The immediate effects of stress, such as a raised heart rate, heightened senses, and increased ability to concentrate, for example, are helpful when we have to compete, avoid an accident, meet a deadline, or give a talk in front of a large group. It's the slow-boiling, long-term stress that, well, can really get under our skin and inflict lasting damage.

The word *stress* as it relates to emotions became part of our everyday vocabulary in the 1950s. Then its use became even more common during the long later decades of the Cold War, an era when fear ruled. Today we continue to use the word to describe anything that disrupts us emotionally — be it the threat of global war or just going to war at work with a difficult colleague.

Since Selye's time, researchers have broken stress down into several subcategories. A key concept that has entered the medical vernacular is what is known as *allostasis* and, in turn, *allostatic load*. Allostasis is another word for "homeostasis," or the body's attempt to maintain physiological balance and equilibrium. Your allostatic load refers to environmental challenges—"wear and tear" on the body. When the load reaches a certain threshold, the body begins efforts to maintain stability (allostasis).

Your allostatic load also refers to the physiological consequences of adapting to chronic stress, including repeated activation of the body's stress-response machinery across many systems—immune, endocrine, and neuronal. Which is why this load can be measured by looking at chemical imbalances in the nervous, hormonal, and immune systems. It can also be measured by monitoring disturbances in the body's day-night cycle (what's called the circadian rhythm, another concept we'll explore later) and, in some cases, by noting changes in the brain's physical structure.

Researchers Bruce McEwen and Eliot Stellar coined the term *allostatic load* in 1993 as a more precise alternative to the generic term *stress*.[3] The main players of the stress response, cortisol and adrenaline (epinephrine), have good and bad sides: they can have either protective or damaging effects on the body, depending on when and in what quantity they are secreted. On the one hand, they are essential for adaptation and maintenance of homeostasis, but if they are flowing for a prolonged period or needed relatively frequently, they increase allostatic load and can accelerate disease processes. The allostatic load, in this case, becomes more harmful than helpful as chemical imbalances and physiological disturbances take root in the body.

Stress is a good thing, at least from an evolutionary and survivalist perspective. It serves an important function: to protect us from real danger by equipping us with the means to either escape a life-threatening situation or face it head-on. But our physical response doesn't change according to the type or magnitude of a perceived threat. The body's stress response is the same whether you're facing a life-or-death stressor, a packed to-do list, or an argument with a friend or family member. To really understand the impact of stress on your skin, we first need to look at what happens inside your body when it senses stress.

THE BIOLOGY OF STRESS

Your body pulses twenty-four hours a day to the rhythmic tune of hormones. And I'm not just talking about the well-known sex hormones testosterone and estrogen. Our hormonal (endocrine) system is highly complex and self-regulated. Dozens of hormones are at work every moment to get certain physiologic functions accomplished, including those going on in your skin. Hormones control a lot of what you feel physically—be it hungry, full, sleepy, energetic, hot, or cold. Among their many jobs is to help transport substances through membranes, manage the rate of certain chemical reactions, regulate water and electrolyte balance, and keep a check on blood pressure. They manage development, growth, reproduction, and overall behavior. It helps to think of them as the body's little messengers. These messengers are produced in certain parts of the body—such as the thyroid, in the neck; the adrenal glands, which sit atop the kidneys; and the pituitary gland, deep in your brain—and reach target tissues and organs in other parts of the body through the blood or other bodily fluids. Once at their destinations, they can do their jobs, acting to modify structures and functions. Hormones are part of every major system in the body, from your reproductive system to your digestive, immune, urinary, respiratory, cardiovascular, nervous, muscular, and skeletal systems.

Stress of any kind, be it from chronic sleep deprivation or the pain of going through a divorce, can do a number on your endocrine system. And if, as a result, your hormones are not optimally balanced, or they are not working effectively, you will eventually begin to notice it. Your skin will not escape these challenges. Any of the Big Four skin conditions can be part of this picture. Note that hormonal disturbances can also be a result of your age and stage of life, such as puberty, pregnancy, and menopause. Hormones also can get thrown out of whack under the influence of a disease (e.g., diabetes and hypothyroidism) or an invading pathogen that changes your body's biology. As you now know, an imbalance in your intestinal microbiome can lead to gut dysfunction, which also affects your body's hormonal status.

Let's consider in more detail the series of events that occurs when the body encounters stress. Some of the hormones involved were mentioned in previous pages, but here I'll help you gain a better understanding of how they can have a direct impact on your appearance.

The HPA Axis

A clear and defined cascade of events happens when the body senses stress. First the brain sends a distress signal to the adrenal glands that results in the release of adrenaline, also called epinephrine. Your heart rate increases as blood is diverted away from things like digestion and directed to your muscles in case you need to flee. If the surge in adrenaline is fierce enough, it will pull blood from the skin and face, too. As the threat abates, so does the response, and your body eventually returns to normal. But if danger persists and your stress response intensifies with no end in sight, then your body enters another state, one in which a specialized team of hormones is called in to help manage things. This series of events takes place along what's called the HPA axis, short for hypothalamic–pituitary–adrenal axis.

The hypothalamus is a small but key governing region of the brain that has a vital role in controlling many bodily functions, including the release of hormones from the pea-size pituitary gland, housed inside it. The hypothalamus is often referred to as the seat of our emotions because it directs much of our emotional processing. The moment you feel nervous, anxious, or overwhelmed, the hypothalamus releases a chemical called corticotropin-releasing hormone (CRH) to start a chain reaction that ends with cortisol flowing into your bloodstream from the adrenals (other substances are also released, including inflammatory cytokines, but I'm going to keep this simple).

You're already familiar with cortisol, the body's main stress hormone, which aids in that famous fight-or-flight response. But because it's responsible for protecting you during times of stress, it also controls how your body processes carbohydrates, fats, and proteins. Cortisol can increase your appetite, promote fat storage, and break down materials that can be used for quick forms of energy. For this reason, exposure to excess cortisol over time can lead to increased belly fat (the worst kind to have), bone loss, a suppressed immune system, fatigue, and a heightened risk of insulin resistance, diabetes, and heart disease.[4] It also is infamous for breaking down certain tissues, including collagen in skin. And it disrupts the formation of new skin, making skin thinner and weaker.

Collagen is the body's most abundant protein. It comprises one-third of the body's total protein, accounts for three-quarters of the dry weight of skin, and is the most prevalent component of the extracellular matrix.[5] So as you can imagine, collagen continuously undergoes a cycle of renewal (including breakdown and repair). In fact it's what makes your skin (and muscles, which are also rich in collagen) particularly adept at repairing cells after damage. Think of the last time you pulled a muscle or burned your skin. Within days, the damaged tissue was well on its way to being fully repaired as the body's turnover factory went to work. This turnover engine, however, starts to sputter with age. This means you're more vulnerable to tissue damage, and recovery can take longer. And when the body experiences such stress, it exposes you to increased cortisol levels. While cortisol's role in priming the body to defend itself against attack would be wonderful if the threat were short-lived and easily resolved, the attack of our modern-day lifestyles is unrelenting.

The Body's Counterattack

The body's counterattack on stress does not just involve surges in stress hormones such as cortisol and the subsequent breakdown of tissues such as collagen. In addition, two other players are often involved in direct skin damage: inflammation and oxidation.

Inflammation, which I talked about in chapter 1, is the body's protective mechanism against harmful stimuli. It's the process by which our bodies can effectively kill an invader or deal with an illness. But, like cortisol, it has a downside—over time, it can cause everything from skin problems such as acne and rosacea to autoimmune disorders and depression.

Oxidation results from the action of free radicals—a term you're probably already familiar with. Free radicals are the biological equivalent of wayward bullets. They are indeed radical and free—highly reactive forms of oxygen that can damage cell membranes and other structures in the body. But their wrath is especially brutal on the skin. Free radicals can come from anywhere—from inside our bodies, where they are produced as part of our normal physiological processes, to pollution and UV rays, just two of the external sources of stress on the skin.

The scientific study of the impact of stress on the body from the inside out, and even the outside in, has made tremendous advances since 1998, when Harvard University researchers conducted a collaborative study with several hospitals in the Boston area.[6] It was designed to better understand mind–body interactions and their effect on skin.

The researchers set out to look at the way various external forces—from massage and aromatherapy to social isolation—influence our state of mind. And what they found confirmed what many in the scientific community have known anecdotally for centuries: our state of mind has a profound impact on our health *and appearance*.

They named their discovery the NICE (neuro-immuno-cutaneous-endocrine) network. It helps to think of it as a giant interactive network composed of your nervous system, immune system, skin, and endocrine (hormonal) system. These are all intimately connected through a complex web of biochemicals that speak to one another—from pleasurable endorphins to proinflammatory compounds.

Dozens of other studies have since confirmed the powerful interplay between psychology and biology, or, put simply, the mind–body relationship (skin included). The brain and skin communicate upon exposure to psychological stress or environmental stress factors. And we've come to learn that the body has more than one stress response system that has outward effects. There's one that can occur locally *in the skin*. That's right: the skin is an endocrine organ itself and contains its own personal HPA-like axis.

The Skin's Personalized HPA

Emotional and psychological stress have long been linked to virtually every type of skin condition, from dermatitis to acne, psoriasis, itchy and red skin, and aging.[7] How is this possible? While this area of study is still evolving, we do have a foundation of knowledge to help us understand the relationship. As I just described, albeit simply, upon the brain's perception of psychological stress, the hypothalamic-pituitary-adrenal axis is activated, releasing certain chemicals (mostly stress hormones) as well as an immune response to help the body deal with the "threat." This can result in signals to the skin that translate to inflammatory conditions. But the same response can occur locally in the skin, releasing the same chemicals—hormones and endorphins included. The skin can respond to stress all on its own without the brain's help. Remember: not only does it have its own stress response system, it has its own immune system as well.

All this ultimately means that our skin can instigate reactions that cause all manner of skin conditions. Moreover, the messages that come blasting out from the skin locally, and possibly in combination with stress messages originating from the central nervous system, can have a direct effect on the production of collagen and elastin, those beauty-promoting fibers. Certain stress responses will slow down or even stop their growth.

So when you experience inflammation in the skin, it could be coming not only from the brain's signaling, via the central HPA, but also from the skin itself. Environmental factors such as UV light, heat, cold, pollution, infection, irritants, allergens, high or low humidity, and free radicals are also capable of inducing a skin stress response. In turn, the skin's stress response system can activate the central HPA and add to the body's overall stress load.

Our "Allergic Reactions" to Stress

Our skin can have an almost allergic reaction to stressors. The skin contains cells called mast cells—a type of white blood cell that, when activated by stress, releases certain stress-related hormones, such as histamines. Histamines, which are located near nerve endings and blood vessels, are central players in allergies and inflammation. They are the catalysts behind conditions such as asthma and hay fever. They are also implicated in many skin disorders and diseases. A number of biochemicals can activate mast cells, but the one that gets their attention the most is CRH (corticotropin-releasing hormone). In fact mast cells may be the richest source of CRH outside the brain. How so? Mast cells can make CRH on their own!

Once these mast cells are triggered biochemically, they can stimulate reactions that result in a spectrum of skin conditions—or they can exacerbate existing ones. The originating trigger can be any number of things that the body translates as stress: exposure to pollution or UV light, a strong emotion, pain, free radicals, or extreme temperatures. Don't forget that signals between your skin and brain go both ways, so a relatively minor skin issue (e.g., a mosquito bite or mild sunburn) might tell your brain to keep the stress levels up, which means you get stuck in a cycle of inflammation and irritation. And I hate to break it to you, but when stress causes inflammation in skin, the skin forms more nerve fibers, which makes it even more sensitive. A vicious cycle can set in!

It helps to think of this bidirectional communication between your central nervous system and skin, as well as within your skin itself, as your own personal Wi-Fi system. The dialogue is carried through *peptides*—small chains of amino acids that facilitate cellular communication. *Neuropeptides* originate in the nervous system and brain, including the peripheral nerve endings in skin. There's one neuropeptide in particular that gets a lot of play in research circles: substance P. This well-known chemical promotes pain (hence the *P*) in the body and can increase sebum production. This is why it is often implicated in acne. As we'll see later on, certain strains of probiotics have been shown to help control substance P, making them a useful tool in controlling acne. Substance P has also been shown to be a factor in depression and anxiety, which are often associated with acne.

Here's what transpires: when your body senses stress, your nerves respond—especially nerve endings in the skin. They send out substance P, then receptors in your skin react by sharing that message with other cells, telling them how to function. You have experienced this chain of events when you feel a deep emotion and it shows up on your face. If you're embarrassed, you blush; when you're exuberant, your skin is likely to glow; when frightened, your skin can change color in an instant.

What's going on locally on your skin depends on how your skin "thinks" and "feels." Those environmental stress factors can send substance P and other peptides rushing to your skin. The skin aims to defend itself and marshal its repair staff. Skin's production of collagen and elastin reflects these peptides' activity. If your skin is under too much environmental stress, your collagen and elastin factories will shut down. Conversely, if your skin is free of stressors and supported healthfully, those production lines can run smoothly and contribute to youthful-looking skin.

My hope is that you're now realizing that your skin issues are much more than "skin deep." The good news is that while the mind can act as an incredibly powerful weapon for inflicting bodily harm, it's also, with the right information, a profound resource for reversing these conditions and promoting luminous skin. We'll get to the tools for transforming skin through the mind in part II, but for now, let's go to treating skin topically.

CHAPTER 4

Face Value

What You Know About Skin Care Is Wrong

I have a confession to make. My skin isn't perfect now, and it wasn't perfect when I was twenty. You already know I love being outside. Well, I didn't always practice "safe sun." Sometimes I went outside with baby oil on so I could get a bronze tan like the ones some of my friends had. Did it work? No, it did not, because I am fair with blond hair, blue eyes, and freckles! I also didn't know that much about sunscreen as a kid, and neither did my mom, but after a few scalp burns, I began rocking a hat, colored zinc-oxide sunscreen, and long sleeves over my swimsuit.

Fast-forward many years, during which I gained a lot of wisdom and experience. I no longer use baby oil. I now know that a white T-shirt offers an SPF of about 5, so it isn't a solution. I know how to balance my love of the sun with my love of healthy skin. I practice what I preach. I've tackled the premature aging of my skin from so much sun exposure as well as psoriasis and intermittent adult acne, which I have gotten under control based on the principles in this book. Rest assured that I take care of my skin following the same guidelines I'm giving you in these pages!

I've come a long way since my overly sun-drenched youth in terms of how I treat my skin daily. Most of my patients are surprised when I order them to stop washing their faces so often, throw out their loofahs, and never again squirt an antimicrobial gel into their hands, even if they are in a public place where germs lurk. When they come to me, the majority of them would score poorly if I were to quiz them about good skin care. But you, on the other hand, will be able to ace the test once you get to the end of this chapter. I'm debunking the myths and giving you the secrets to skin care.

It's been estimated that by 2020, the value of the global skin-care market will reach $179 billion (up from $130 billion in 2015).[1] Among the driving forces cited is heightened skin-care awareness. People—both young and old—are more informed about the value of taking care of their skin, especially in an era when skin-cancer rates are soaring and when selfies are the norm. Thanks to scientific advances, skin care is no longer just about topical cleansers and moisturizers. It is also about topical probiotics and serums that protect the skin's microbiome.

As you are learning, skin is much more than a physical barrier. It serves as a thermostat, a parasol, a shock absorber, an insulator, a wound healer, and a critical part of our immune system. This last role is paramount: when we think of our immune system, we tend to think of white blood cells and lymph tissue, but it's becoming increasingly accepted that beneficial species of microorganisms found on the surface of and deep within the skin are integral parts of the immune system. And when the balance of those colonies is thrown off, or when the skin's barrier is compromised, trouble ensues. (Much as the intestinal wall can become "leaky," so can the skin, leading to inflammation and an aggravation of the immune system.)

As you are also learning, human skin is a veritable ecosystem comprising life forms we cannot see with the naked eye, including bacteria, fungi, and viruses. Most of these microbes are either beneficial or harmless, but some have been linked to skin conditions such as acne, rosacea, psoriasis, and eczema. Investigating the variability of microbial communities across different skin sites has been key to understanding, for example, why psoriasis tends to affect dry, exposed areas such as the elbows and knees, whereas eczema commonly develops in moist areas such as the bends of the arms and legs. Skin is also a factory that produces, in addition to sweat, vitamin D, hormones, oils, wax, and pigments — substances we need for survival.

Skin is a unique organ in that it has multiple responsibilities. It's arguably the most dynamic, hardworking organ of all, which is why supporting and maintaining the gut-brain-skin axis is critical. All the creams in the world won't work if you don't correct what's going wrong from the inside out. This doesn't dismiss the role of cleansers and moisturizers or the usefulness of dermatologists and prescription products when necessary. As much as I want you to take care of your skin from the inside out, I also want you to treat it well from the outside in. It is the only way to realize your goal of truly beautiful skin.

Before we dive into our skin-care plan, let's have a more in-depth look at the makeup of our skin — its layers and key structures, how it functions, what it needs to heal and renew itself, and why it's key to our survival.

ANATOMY OF THE SKIN YOU'RE IN

Skin's main job is, not surprisingly, to be one of your body's biggest gatekeepers to the outside world. It is also the means through which we experience the wonderful sense of touch. And it's one of the few organs that can regenerate itself. As skin discards dead cells, it grows new ones to replace them. Every four to five weeks, you've made yourself a new outer coating, so to speak.

From a structural standpoint, skin is a multilayered organ. And from a mechanical perspective, it helps to think of skin as resembling a manufacturing plant—a building several stories high. And because it manufactures a lot of things, it needs supplies, sources of energy, employees, and an efficient assembly line. Although skin appears from the outside to be made up of one type of cell, it is far from that. Skin needs an enormous array of compounds—including proteins, amino acids, vitamins, trace minerals, antioxidants, fats, water, and even sugar (in healthful amounts!)—to perform all its functions. To stay safe and sound, it must keep its structures intact and healthy. Skin is a high-maintenance machine that needs more attention as you age because, like any piece of machinery, it loses some of its performance ability with time and constant (24-7) use—and the loss is even greater if you don't maintain it.

The Factory's Basement

At the base of your skin's "building" is a layer of fat. We call it subcutaneous (below-the-skin) fat, and it provides protective padding, insulation from heat and cold, and energy storage. During the natural aging process, your skin's fat layer shrinks, which is why old folks can feel heat and cold more acutely than young people and their cheeks are often less plump.

Your skin's basement is also where your sweat glands begin, branching upward toward the surface. Our sweat glands help filter out water and electrolytes, such as salt. They're a critical part of your personal air-conditioning system, working so you don't overheat. As sweat evaporates, your body can cool down and return to its ideal core temperature (98.6 degrees Fahrenheit).

Lymph and blood vessels also make up the skin's foundation. These important vessels play many roles, from transmitting messages and delivering nutrients to clearing out waste and transporting substances needed to address problems such as open cuts, sores, and infections.

The Factory's Middle Floors

The two-layered dermis is the largest part of your skin, accounting for about 90 percent of its mass. In addition to housing blood and lymph vessels and nerve endings, it provides architectural elements that add structure, elasticity, and resiliency. The dermis's infrastructure is supported by a type of tough connective tissue—a mesh of collagen and elastin fibers produced constantly by nearby cells called fibroblasts. As with so many other aspects of the body as it ages, production slows down over time.

The rich layers of the dermis are home to many other important things that help keep skin youthful. The fact that it's composed of about 60 percent water and a gel-like collection of various molecules that nourish and trap moisture says a lot about its role. This is also where your sebaceous, or oil, glands reside. The oil glands, as you can probably guess, produce that oily, moisture-loving substance called sebum, which helps keep skin soft and supple. Of course this same sebum can trigger acne when too much is produced and clogs pores.

Hair follicles originate in the dermis, and glycosaminoglycans (GAGs for short) also roam there. GAGs are water-loving polysaccharides (a type of carbohydrate) that help moisturize skin and bolster collagen. The dominating GAG that surrounds the collagen-elastin mesh network is hyaluronic acid, which is found in a lot of topical products today. Hyaluronic acid binds the collagen-elastin mesh together, helping keep the skin hydrated. Levels of hyaluronic acid decline as you age, so your skin becomes less pliable and prone to dryness.

When we watch someone visibly age, either naturally or prematurely as a result of various factors such as exposure to UV radiation, environmental pollution, and poor dietary choices, most of the changes we see take place in the dermis. Fibroblasts decrease in number, leaving you with less collagen. If you've "used" your skin a lot—smiling, laughing, frowning, raising an eyebrow—this will have an impact and result in more wrinkling. Such lines will be further deepened by that subcutaneous fat loss.

Age also comes with hormonal changes that can affect skin. A combination of estrogen loss after menopause as well as a slowdown of oil and sweat production leads to drier skin. Blood vessels, vital for delivering nutrients and moisture and getting rid of cellular waste, also decline in number, which can lead to dull-looking skin. If the to-and-fro of nutrients and waste is not as active as it was, the skin cannot renew itself as well or remain properly nourished and hydrated, and the signs of aging set in. Sun damage and smoking will exacerbate the situation. UV rays cause blood-vessel walls to thicken. Those vessels can become visible when they dilate and show up as tiny red threads just below the skin's surface in the dermis. You already know that smoking is bad for your skin (and everything else). Tobacco smoke, in fact, affects skin from the inside, via the toxic by-products that travel through the bloodstream and reach dermal cells, as well as from the outside, where epidermal tissues (see below) are directly exposed to tobacco smoke. "Smoker's skin" is easy to spot, as it's often discolored and appears advanced in age. Smoking literally suffocates your skin from the inside out and outside in, limiting its access to much-needed nutrients, hydration, and oxygen.

The Upper Factory Floor

Now the elevator has reached the epidermis—skin's outer layer, which is exposed to light and the outside world. The epidermis draws in water, light, and heat while it deflects dirt, germs, and toxins. Special cells called keratinocytes are abundant in the epidermis. Keratinocytes, as their name implies, produce keratin, which is the same tough waterproofing protein that makes up hair and fingernails. Born at the base of the epidermis, keratinocytes flatten out as they move up to the surface, where they die and help form a barrier. This layer of dead cells is known as the stratum corneum, which is the layer we can see and touch.

Present in all layers of the epidermis except the stratum corneum are soldierlike cells called Langerhans cells. These cells are a critical part of your skin's immune system, because they detect foreign substances. So important are they to your immunity that they are also found in your respiratory, digestive, and urogenital tracts. But rather than act as alarmists and foment strong reactions to infection and inflammation, they are known to turn the volume down on immune reactions and help keep the peace. As you know, skin is at the mercy of the environment all day long, but most challenges to skin from the environment are not in fact harmful and do not warrant an immune response. Your Langerhans constantly work to stop the immune system from acting like an oversensitive toddler throwing a tantrum. In 2011, it was discovered that these cells share a unique relationship with the skin's microbiome.[2] Not only do these important immune cells in the outer layers of our skin keep us from experiencing unnecessary immune reactions that can trigger skin disorders, they also stop the immune system from attacking friendly bacteria. They help the skin's microbial community maintain the right balance for optimal health and, in turn, appearance. Later in the book, I'll reveal how one strain of bacteria (when taken as an oral probiotic) may help protect your Langerhans.

The cells that determine your skin color—melanocytes—also reside in the epidermis. These cells produce melanin, the pigment that protects skin from too much ultraviolet light by darkening (i.e., tanning) it after repeated UV exposure, which can damage skin's DNA. But as any fair-skinned person will tell you, some types of melanin are too light to provide any decent UV protection. People who have them, like me, burn easily. The number of melanocytes in skin decreases with age, which means the older you are the more susceptible you become to

UV rays. The epidermis in general is prone to discoloration as it ages and reflects its lifetime of exposure to the environment. The older you are, the more likely you are to develop brown spots and even some white spots as well as a pale overall appearance. And as that top layer thins over the decades, it becomes a less effective barrier to potential invaders and toxins from the outside world as well as less effective at trapping moisture.

BEAUTY BUGS

The year 2013 was a game changer in my field. After my 2011 paper described how skin's appearance is partly rooted in the gut and the gut's microbiome, other researchers have shown the power of skin's microclimate—mainly its local microbiome—and published some staggering findings.[3] As with so many things in the scientific world, it can take only a single definitive and well-executed study to turn conventional wisdom on its head. We used to think the skin's microbiome flourished mainly on the surface and that the deeper dermal layers were relatively sterile. We know better now, thanks to some inquiring scientists from the University of California at San Diego who dug a little deeper.[4] Turns out that microbes reside all the way down to the subcutaneous fat layer. This is where the most intimate communication between the microbiome and our immune system takes place.

Among the skin's trillions of organisms, bacteria dominate, as they do in the gut. There are more than one thousand different bacterial species, eighty different fungi species (by some estimates), plenty of viruses, and a few mites. Our SALT (skin-associated lymphoid tissue) is highly active. You can think of your SALT as a local lymph system built into your skin: it contains lymphocytes that help defend the body against harmful foreign particles and debris. In fact each square centimeter of skin contains more than a million bacteria living in commensal symbiosis, and more than a million lymphocytes. A one-to-one bug-to-lymphocyte ratio.

The skin's microbiome is also similar to the gut's in the sense that it tends to remain relatively stable over time, but it does vary depending on its location (or ecological niche). The flora in your armpits, for example, will be different from what's found on your back. Colonies also change depending on the amount of light, the pH level, and whether the area is moist, warm, dry, hairy, or oily. Age and gender also play a role, varying the microbial composition. An active pubescent girl will have a very different microbiome from that of a relatively sedentary postmenopausal woman or middle-aged man.

We are just beginning to explore and understand the skin's microbiome and how its actions both at the skin's surface as well as deep beneath its outer layers affect the rest of the body. It's likely that the closest communication between the skin microbiome and the general immune system takes place far down in the skin's subcutaneous chambers, which has inspired some researchers to call the microbiome of skin's deep layers the "host indigenous microbiome."[5] New research is also uncovering how closely a person's microbial profile—the overall balance of bacteria on his or her skin—correlates with various skin disorders. At the Microbiology Society's annual conference in 2017, Dr. Emma Barnard, a researcher in the Department of Molecular and Medical Pharmacology at the UCLA School of Medicine, presented eye-opening work done by her team in this regard.[6] She showed that the presence or absence of particular bacterial strains is an important factor in acne development and skin health. The bacterium *Propionibacterium acnes* (*P. acnes*) has long been associated with acne, but since it's the most prevalent and abundant species in the follicles of both clear-skinned individuals and those with acne, its role has not been well understood. Could it be that various strains of *P. acnes* have various effects on the skin and thus factor into whether or not one suffers from acne? It appears so.

Barnard's team used over-the-counter pore-cleansing strips to obtain skin follicle samples from seventy-two individuals: thirty-eight with acne and thirty-four without (granted, this was a very small study, but it nonetheless provided new insights and opened the door to previously uncharted territory). The team then used a nifty technique called DNA shotgun sequencing analysis to identify and compare the makeup of the two groups' skin microbiomes. They also repeated the experiment in an additional ten individuals. Remarkably, the researchers pinpointed fine genetic differences between the *P. acnes* strains found in the two clinical groups. In the group without acne, the bacterial community was found to be enriched with genes associated with bacterial metabolism, which are thought to be important in preventing harmful bacteria from colonizing the skin.

In the other group, by contrast—the one suffering from acne—the bacteria contained higher levels of genes associated with acne, including those relating to the production and transport of proinflammatory compounds, such as bacterial toxins that are potentially harmful to the skin. Dr. Barnard's conclusion reflects the new thinking in dermatology, which extends far beyond treating acne: "Understanding the bacterial community on the skin is important for the development of personalized treatments in acne. Instead of killing all bacteria, including the beneficial ones, we should focus on shifting the balance toward a healthy microbiota by targeting harmful bacteria or enriching beneficial bacteria."[7] This concept could be extended to other skin conditions, too.

A healthy skin microbiome serves multiple functions. First, it protects against infection in much the same way a good gut microbiome does—by crowding out the overgrowth of pathogenic (bad) organisms. The skin's microbes also create an acidic environment (i.e., one with a pH level of about 5), which naturally inhibits the growth of pathogens that prefer a more alkaline, less acidic environment. (Note: bad bacteria tend to do better at a more alkaline pH—and some soaps have a pH of about 10!)

Second, there is an ongoing conversation between the skin's local immune system and its microbiome, which helps control inflammation. When the microbiome is out of line, the immune system can release various antimicrobial peptides, such as cathelicidin, to help balance things out. Likewise, our good bacterial residents can inhibit the release of inflammatory compounds from the immune system. In this way, the microbiome controls the skin's immune system, just as the gut's microbiome helps regulate our systemic immune system. The microbiome also aids in wound healing, limits exposure to allergens and UV radiation, minimizes oxidative damage, and keeps the skin plump and moist. That's a lot of tasks for a bunch of invisible little bugs! (I'll go into more details about these facts in the next chapter.)

Recall that an infant's early life exposure to bacterial colonies during the birth process can help establish his or her gut microbiome and have lifelong health repercussions. The same is true with the skin's microbiome. New research conducted on mice suggests that in early infancy, the skin's developing microbiome is not attacked by the body's main immune system because it is involved in establishing a so-called tolerance.[8] The body's immune system learns to accept and live with the skin's microbiome, which researchers hypothesize may ultimately reduce the incidence of autoimmune diseases later in life. The immune system does not get confused between what's truly foreign and harmful and what's part of the "self."

Anything that damages the skin's microbiome in infancy, such as the routine use of broad-spectrum antibiotics, may compromise the development of this tolerance, allowing for the development of autoimmunity, among other health challenges. Kids who suffer from chronic ear infections, for example, can find themselves taking antibiotic after anti-biotic throughout many years of their early development. These power-ful drugs wreak havoc not only on the gut's microbiome but also on the skin's. Sometimes those changes are temporary, and the skin and gut flora can go back to "normal" (everyone's normal will be different). But if antibiotic use is frequent enough, it can alter a child's microbial profile in a profound way and theoretically predispose him or her to future autoimmune diseases and allergies. If you think this describes you, or if you suffer from an autoimmune condition today that could have its roots in a confused immune system early in life, my program will help you optimize your body's overall ability to function properly.

As I hinted in previous chapters, there is something to be said for getting a little bit dirty once in a while. If you suffer from allergies, or if a family member suffers from them, then you may have heard about the hygiene hypothesis. In 1989, the British epidemiologist David Strachan was the first to suggest that exposure to infections during childhood would provide a good defense against allergies in later life.[9] An allergy is, in fact, the immune system stepping out of line by perceiving a harmless substance as a major attack. It is now well documented that people who grew up in an overly sanitized environment (as is often the case in developed, industrialized nations, especially in upper-middle-class communities) have a much higher risk of suffering from autoim-mune and allergic conditions. Without proper challenges to the immune system early in life—via exposure to infectious agents, friendly microorganisms, and even parasites—the immune system doesn't develop properly, increasing susceptibility to allergic reactions. It is as if lack of early life exposure suppresses the natural development of the immune system and creates "glitches," if you will, in what would otherwise be a highly resilient and well-functioning system. This explains why kids who grow up on a traditional farm (not an industrial one) build up strong immune systems that fight true pathogens (e.g., parasites), while children who live in the proverbial urban bubble and are protected from germs can end up with confused immune systems that end up attacking harmless molecules—and, in the form of auto-immune diseases, even the self.[10]

The Connection Between Cleanliness and Allergies

In dermatology, we hear a lot about what's called the atopic march (sometimes referred to as the allergic march), which could be related to the hygiene hypothesis. We often see a natural progression—a "march"—of diagnoses in early life: first atopic dermatitis (eczema) in the first six months of life, then asthma beginning between the ages of two and four, and finally allergic rhinitis (hay fever) in school-age children. Sometimes food allergies also emerge. A steep rise in the number of people, usually children, who suffer from one or more of these conditions has resulted in investigations that led scientists to determine that excessive cleanliness in a child's environment is partly to blame. Future research will bear this out, but one thing is clear: people who are obsessed with germ- and bacteria-free living are setting themselves up not only for serious skin disorders but for other health conditions as well.

Coming up, we'll look at how you can optimally take care of your skin's microbiome. The most egregious insults to it are all the harsh soaps, sanitizers, cleansers, and antimicrobials on the market today. The hygiene hypothesis is not just about how excess cleanliness and exposure to antibiotics increase the risk for many illnesses, allergies, and autoimmune issues by damaging the gut microbiome. By logical extension, it applies to skin as well: when you overcleanse, oversani-tize, and/or expose it to too many antibiotics (which kill the good guys along with the bad guys), you open yourself up to an imbalanced skin microbiome (creating "skin dysbiosis") and a whole host of skin conditions.

I think that's enough basic skin biology. Now you have a frame-work of knowledge about skin's multilayered complexities so you can appreciate its hardworking powers. Skin and its microbial inhabitants comprise a highly dynamic organ that does a lot for us. It can withstand a lot—it has to, given its constant exposure to the outside world. But it can also be easily compromised when it's not taken care of properly.

Let me ask you this: when was the last time you saw (or used) a hand sanitizer? Do you have one in your purse? Keep them in your car? Feel dirty or perhaps even "naked" without the cool sensation on your hands a few times a day? These ubiquitous gel, foam, and liquid solutions are quick and convenient when you don't have running water and soap around. But they are not only toxic to the skin, its barrier function, and its microbial collaborators, they are also dangerous. Studies show that they don't reduce or prevent infections as effectively as does washing with gentle hand soap and water, and some of their ingredients have even been shown to do more damage than we realized. Triclosan, for example, is a common ingredient in hygiene products (check your toothpaste), though it has been banned from most soaps. Why? According to the FDA, triclosan may lead to hormonal disruptions and cause bacteria to adapt to its antimicrobial properties, thus creating more antibiotic-resistant strains.[11] It makes me wonder: what other ingredients are in these hand sanitizers that are harmful but not banned yet?

Don't get me wrong: sanitation and cleanliness have dramatically improved our health over the past century, and regular hand washing is a big part of that. But now we are overdoing it with chronic exposure to harsh chemicals and a belief that "more is better" when it comes to cleanliness everywhere on our bodies. That just is not true. To prove it, let's turn to the science of probiotics on skin health—both orally and topically. This is where the research speaks for itself and is truly exciting.

CHAPTER 5

The Power in Going Pro

Why Probiotics Are the New Antibiotics

Humans have had an epic, often tempestuous history with bacteria. In the fourteenth century, the bubonic plague (the Black Death), caused by the bacterium *Yersinia pestis,* obliterated nearly one-third of the population of Europe over the course of just five years. (Back in the Middle Ages no one knew what caused the plague: rumors abounded, from divine punishment to the pus in acne blemishes.) In 2014, it was estimated that the global toll of bacteria-related deaths will reach ten million per year by 2050—more than those caused by cancer.[1]

For centuries, we didn't have antibiotics to combat deadly bacterial infections. Nobody even knew bacteria existed until the late-seventeenth-century Dutch tradesman and inquisitive scientist Anton van Leeuwenhoek performed a little self-experimentation by peering through a microscope at his own dental plaque. He called the mysterious single-cell organisms animalcules (literally, "microscopic animals"). Not surprisingly, this observation secured him the title of father of microbiology. Van Leeuwenhoek lived during the century of the scientific revolution. As European explorers ventured west and colonized the Americas, scientific inquiry grew in Europe, and scientists introduced a new understanding of the natural world. By the end of that century, we had logarithms, electricity, calculus, Newton's laws, Galileo's observations, telescopes, and, thanks to Van Leeuwenhoek's inventiveness, more sophisticated microscopes. But it would take another few centuries for us to understand the infectious nature of certain bacteria and discover antibiotics, which is something that really happened by chance.

Antibiotics have saved millions of lives since the early twentieth century, but we now have a different problem. As a result of the profligate use of these powerful drugs over the course of more than fifty years, we've spurred the creation of drug-resistant superbugs. Some have argued that the superbug problem is on a par with climate change in terms of severity. In 2016, the United Nations convened over the matter and pledged to fight antibiotic resistance in a historic agreement. The FDA has begun to ban certain products that contain antimicrobial ingredients for fear they will fuel more resistant strains of bacteria.

The Western world's obsession with hygiene has only worsened the situation. Take a look around you: sanitizer dispensers are everywhere. Soaps in public restrooms are often antimicrobial. Public areas are doused in bleach, and municipal water sources are cleansed with chlorine. Every day, you expose yourself to these chemicals, which are torpedoing your skin and its microbiome. Even daily showers compound your vulnerability. Don't panic: I won't be asking you to stop bathing, but I will be telling you how to do so more safely. There's a lot you can do, including choosing which soaps to use at home and knowing how to avoid the antimicrobials in public venues.

Although many of us still perceive bacteria as agents of death, the time has come to appreciate another side to their purpose in our lives. They are, after all, among the original inhabitants of the earth—beating us by billions of years. While there are some bad bugs out there, there are more good ones that are critical—not detrimental—to a healthful life. Supporting their functionality is the only way to not just win the war against superbugs but also restore our skin health.

Before I highlight what beneficial bacteria can do for our skin, I want to reiterate some important facts so you can grasp how powerful probiotics can be in helping support the body's microbiome. Recall that your microbiome helps control a lot of your physiology, especially your immune system. Through the actions of their surface proteins, which act as antennae and receive messages, and the substances they manufacture, which interact with your own cells, your microbial partners share some of the driver's seat. They speak to your cells all the way down to your DNA. Not only do they collaborate with your body's chief systems, they can also affect the expression of your DNA. I know—it's hard to believe. But your microbiome helps control the expression of genes involved with a variety of physiological factors, including nutrient absorption, energy metabolism, intestinal barrier function, immunity, and inflammation pathways. Which means they also mightily influence whether or not you develop a skin condition.

One more bit of information I want to mention before we move on comes from the work of Dr. Martin Blaser. The director of New York University's Human Microbiome Project, he is among the pioneering researchers who have done extensive work on how the microbiome establishes itself and how disruptions in its early development can result in health challenges later in life. He and his wife, Dr. Maria Gloria Dominguez-Bello, also a researcher at NYU, have documented that children whose microbiomes are somehow compromised or imbalanced go on to have a much higher risk in adulthood for a slew of conditions such as allergies, diabetes, and obesity.[2] Their work in the obesity realm has been particularly interesting and informative for me, because I practice in a field where antibiotics are still the gold standard for many treatments. What Blaser and his colleagues have determined— that chronic overuse of antibiotics can lead to obesity through their impact on the microbiome—will no doubt change how we work.

Blaser effectively demonstrated that when young mice received low doses of antibiotics, they gained 15 percent more body fat than mice that weren't exposed to the antibiotics.[3] In another study, he and his team gave mice a high-fat diet together with antibiotics, leading those mice to become obese.[4] His control group, which ate the same high-fat diet but did not receive antibiotics, did not become obese (antibiotic-treated females fared far worse: they added twice as much body fat as did their untreated female counterparts, who ate the same high-fat diet). Antibiotics change the composition of the gut bacteria to favor strains that encourage weight gain. Dermatologists often use low-dose antibiotics to treat skin conditions such as rosacea over the long term. Considered a safer option compared to high-dose antibiotics because the low dose limits the risks of resistance and other common side effects, they were meant to be more anti-inflammatory than antibacterial. But now that we're seeing what they can do to animals, we are facing a new era. (And yes, this is how farmers fatten up their livestock — using antibiotics not just to kill bad bacteria but also to change the animals' microbiomes and, in turn, their metabolisms so they grow bigger faster.) In the future, it's possible that we will turn only to probiotics to address skin conditions whose treatments once relied primarily on antibiotics.

Probiotic Actions in Your Favor

When it comes to overall skin health, probiotics, whether oral or topical,

- counter harmful bacteria (in the gut and on the skin),
- support barrier function (both in the intestines and on the skin),
- contribute to the regulation of the immune system, both inside and out, by helping control inflammation and oxidative stress, and
- help maintain the working balance of the all-important gut-brain-skin axis.

THE NEXT REVOLUTION IN SKIN MEDICINE

In 2015, I published a paper with my colleague Dr. Mary-Margaret Kober that presented a review of what we know about the effectiveness of probiotics in addressing various skin disorders as well as aging.[5] This added to a growing body of exciting new research about how we can leverage the power of probiotics in treating skin. Human clinical trials and animal studies have provided enough data about probiotics' effects at the molecular level to build a strong, compelling case for their role in treating a wide array of skin conditions while slowing the manifestations of aging—both on the inside and outside! Certain strains are even showing promise with respect to acne, rosacea and redness, and dry skin and eczema.

The question that science is currently trying to address is how probiotics can best be used. In other words, should a topical, oral, or combination approach be recommended? Which strains are most effective? And is it ideal to create a formulation with probiotics and other ingredients that enhance the skin's barrier function? Given where the research stands now and where it's headed, I think it's wise to employ probiotics both orally and topically. Let's look at some of this promising new science, starting with topical probiotics.[6]

TOPICAL PROBIOTIC POWER

Google "probiotics in skin care," and nearly a million results emerge in 0.72 seconds. That's how hot this area is in beauty and wellness circles. Virtually every cosmetics and skin-care company is developing probiotic masks, creams, sprays, and cleansers. Why? Because the science behind what they can do is already scaring those bad bugs away. In many ways, probiotics are the new antibiotics—and the new antidotes to myriad skin issues.

Scientifically speaking, people in R & D circles are determining whether there is a time and place for live organisms (i.e., live bacteria) or whether we need only rely on microbial extracts (such as antimicrobial peptides and natural antibiotics, collectively referred to as "supernatants") to deliver results. I explain it like this: you can either have live bacteria that continue to live and multiply and replace those on the skin or you can grow bacteria in a big jar, then skim off all the good stuff the bacteria have produced as a result of their own metabolism and secreted into their environment—the supernatants. The by-products of bacteria metabolism are increasingly being referred to as postbiotics, and some of these postbiotics have positive effects on human health. Postbiotics can also include heat-killed bacteria, bacterial fragments, and *lysed* bacteria. We can *lyse* bacteria—break them apart either physically, by shaking them, or chemically, by adding a detergentlike ingredient that breaks them apart—then use that *bacterial lysate* in skin-care products. Lysates contain pieces of cell wall along with pieces of DNA, and those pieces might be enough to alter the health of the skin. All this technology is in its explosive beginning, and top scientists at major skin-care companies are exploring how best to utilize it.

Just how do probiotics benefit the skin when applied topically? They mimic the actions of naturally occurring bacteria on your skin in three big ways: (1) they act as a protective shield with calming effects, (2) they provide ammunition against bad bacteria, and (3) they boost skin's innate functionality. These effects ultimately help reduce inflammation, which in turn helps limit flare-ups in skin and prevent premature aging. Let me explain.

PROBIOTICS ACT AS A PROTECTIVE SHIELD WITH CALMING EFFECTS

First, topically applied probiotics cause what's called bacterial interference. Put another way, they protect the skin by interfering with the ability of bad microorganisms to provoke an immune reaction. They essentially "blind" skin cells so they don't see bad microorganisms and other pathogens that can signal an immune response. The bodies of patients with acne and rosacea often perceive the living microorganisms on the skin as foreign and therefore bad and something to attack. So their immune systems jump into action to counter this potential threat, resulting in inflammation, redness, or acne lesions.

I should clarify a few facts about acne and rosacea before moving on. You'll recall that a particular species of bacterium called *P. acnes,* which triggers inflammation, has been implicated as one of the main players in acne. Similarly, a microscopic parasitic mite of the genus *Demodex* can cause rosacea when its numbers proliferate beyond healthful, normal levels. All humans harbor *Demodex;* it is a normal inhabitant of human facial skin. But *Demodex* has often been found in numbers fifteen to eighteen times greater in rosacea patients than in healthy subjects. What's really interesting is that these "bugs" are not infections. It's not like you can just wipe them out using a two-week course of antibiotics. And they are not acting alone. *P. acnes* by itself isn't enough to cause acne, and *Demodex* isn't enough to cause rosacea. They are only part of a complex picture—multiple factors are involved in both skin conditions, including how "revved up" the immune cells in your skin may be.

Topically applied probiotics can actually create a calming environment for skin cells, simply by touching them and connecting with them. Imagine a nurturing caregiver, placing a warm blanket over an anxious child while rubbing his back and telling him that everything will be all right. That soothing, calming environment encourages a child to per-ceive his or her world as less threatening. The same holds true for some strains of probiotics. When they're placed on skin cells, those good bugs calm the parts of the cells that may want to react to a potential threat in the area. These healthy signals produced by the probiotics essentially prevent the skin cells from sending "attack" messages to the immune system that result in acne or rosacea flares. These signals are produced when part of the probiotic binds to part of the skin cell, sending a cas-cade of molecular signals deep into the layers of the skin. They turn on the "happy" signals and turn off the inflammatory torrent of tiny molec-ular messengers. They tell the skin to cease fire. "At ease, troops!"

When cultures of human skin were treated topically with a certain strain of *Lactobacillus paracasei,* for example, scientists were able to show that the probiotic turned the volume down on skin inflammation.[7] It did so by inhibiting substance P, which, you'll recall, is a biomolecule famously tied to inflammation. Substance P is released from nerves and inflammatory cells. Because substance P may amplify inflammation as well as sebum production, controlling it could be a way to treat acne. Clinical trials of topical preparations containing other probiotics have also assessed their effect on acne. One trial involved the facial application of a lotion containing *Enterococcus faecalis* for eight weeks.[8] The scientists noted a 50 percent reduction in the participants' acne compared to peo-ple using a placebo (a lotion without probiotics). Another trial, using *Lactobacillus plantarum,* showed promise, too—decreasing the number and size of acne lesions as well as their redness.[9] *L. plantarum*'s anti-inflammatory effects may also hold promise for reducing rosacea flares.

For the record, we don't really know what causes rosacea, but it typically doesn't appear until adulthood (usually between the ages of thirty and sixty) and is much more common in women than men. It can cause quite a lot of distress, and it doesn't help that conventional treatments, which I mentioned earlier, can exacerbate that unease (no spicy food, no alcohol, and—oh, yeah—don't stress out!). These recommendations often don't provide substantial relief, but probiotics are now leading the way to better results. Masks made with probiotic-rich kefir are proving to be very soothing to skin afflicted by rosacea. And there's a bonus: kefir has the added benefit of containing lactic acid, an antiaging ingredient.

PROBIOTICS PRODUCE SUBSTANCES THAT COMBAT BAD BUGS

Probiotics can help fight harmful bugs, including viruses and fungi, and keep them from triggering inflammation. It's a natural part of a bacterium's survival strategy to make substances that suppress or kill other microbes. Imagine a "good" bacterium shooting tiny little missiles into its environment—your skin. These microbial missiles, also called antimicrobial peptides, can poke holes in "bad" bacteria, causing them to die.

Scientists are currently working to determine which probiotics make the substances that slaughter bad bacteria. I coauthored a paper in 2006 with my mentor at the time, Dr. David Margolis, that was among the first to show how certain substances secreted by bacterial strains can inhibit growth of *P. acnes*.[10] Together we identified one particular strain, *Streptococcus salivarius,* that could effectively combat acne. *S. salivarius* is a prominent component of the microbiome in the mouth and throat and secretes what's called a bacteriocinlike inhibitory substance (BLIS) capable of keeping tabs on *P. acnes*. In addition to their antimicrobial activity, *S. salivarius* bacterial cells themselves inhibit a number of inflammatory pathways, thus making them an important player in immunity. You can thank your *S. salivarius* colonies for helping you avoid ear and throat infections caused by bad bacteria.

My fascination with *S. salivarius* started under the guidance of Dr. Margolis in my med-school days, after I read about Dr. John Tagg, a microbiologist from New Zealand who wanted to find a better way to support throat health in children after he suffered from his own throat conditions as a child.[11] He found that some strains of *S. salivarius* could produce antimicrobial peptides that kill off bad strains of bacteria in the throat, such as the one that causes strep throat (technically, *Streptococcus pyogenes,* also known as group A streptococcus). Dr. Tagg's work intrigued me so much that I wanted to see if this species could also help fight acne (remember, I was a microbiology nut). In fact what I did was go from fraternity house to fraternity house at the University of Pennsylvania collecting samples. I'd swab the tongues and inner cheeks of undergrad frat boys at parties! I then grew and tested the collected strains in a laboratory. Lo and behold I found some specific strains of *S. salivarius* that were amazingly powerful inhibitors of *P. acnes!* They produced little missiles that could stop *P. acnes* in its tracks. This work is what eventually led to my patented BLIS technology for treating acne.[12]

The rise of resistant bacterial pathogens has made this a significant discovery. The *P. acnes* species is getting too smart. It has determined how to avoid eradication, usually through genetic mutations that render it resistant to current therapies. Many commonly used antibiotic treatments are becoming useless because bacteria have essentially managed to revolt, changing in ways that make them impenetrable to our arsenal of drugs. This is already well documented in acne patients harboring resistant *P. acnes* strains. Their acne is totally unaffected by the medications we like to prescribe (in other words, antibiotic lotions that miraculously clear skin in time for the prom are not even making a dent in some teenage skin these days). So we're forced to think of other strategies. What's more, when a patient is using, say, a topical antibiotic for acne, everyone in the house is more prone to carrying resistant strains of bacteria on the skin and in the gut! It can become a self-perpetuating, vicious cycle that leaves everyone more vulnerable and less healthy. And it gets worse: people who use antibiotics to treat acne are twice as likely to develop upper-respiratory-tract infections as people with acne who are not on antibiotics.

The bad-bug-killing power of some bacterial strains extends to other skin conditions as well. Since my work with *S. salivarius,* other researchers have documented certain strains' ability to keep the skin's microbiome in check. Richard Gallo and his colleagues from the University of California at San Diego, for example, have discovered that certain strains of *Staphylococcus,* which naturally lives on human skin (and in our noses and mouths), produce chemicals that kill the bad type of staph — *Staphylococcus aureus.*[13] *S. aureus* can cause severe skin infections and even death when strains become resistant to traditional antibiotics. *S. aureus* was the species that British chemist Alexander Fleming was studying when he discovered antibiotics, in 1928. It is a common member of the skin's family of microbes, but it's especially abundant on people who suffer from eczema.

We don't currently know the exact mechanism for the association between too much *S. aureus* and eczema, but scientists such as Gallo are suggesting that *S. aureus* could at least partly drive the symptoms of eczema, mainly by causing inflammation and triggering allergic reactions. On the other hand, two other strains of staph bacteria — namely *Staphylococcus hominis* (called A9) and *Staphylococcus epidermidis* — can effectively suppress the growth of their evil twin, *S. aureus,* including the more evil drug-resistant versions that we know as methicillin-resistant *S. aureus,* or MRSA. It is thought now that drug-resistant microbes such as MRSA are partly to blame for the ten million people who die each year around the world from infections.

These scientists cleverly furthered their experiments by creating a probiotic cream containing these heroic ingredients and testing it on people with eczema. And amazingly, the subjects' levels of *S. aureus* fell by more than 90 percent. In two people, the culprit bacteria disappeared entirely. In a similar but unrelated study, German scientists identified a microbe called *Staphylococcus lugdunensis* ("lugdunin"), which also thrives in our noses and produces a chemical that specifically kills *S. aureus*.[14] The world awaits more such findings with other strains.

These groundbreaking studies are good news. They signal the start of a new antibiotic era — one in which we look to our own microbial companions to defend our health. Soon we'll know even more about which strains pack the most powerful antimicrobial punch to help keep certain skin conditions at bay and improve skin health.

PROBIOTICS BOOST SKIN'S FUNCTION

The evidence is mounting on the power of topical probiotics in boosting skin's overall functionality as it ages and deals with exposure to damaging elements such as UV radiation. As you can imagine, UV radiation is considered the strongest precipitator of extrinsic aging. As we get older, our body's defense mechanisms grow weaker, including those in the skin that combat free-radical production. If we can't quench free radicals, they will damage cellular structures, including DNA, fats, and proteins such as collagen. Turns out that many probiotics produce substances that not only have antibiotic effects but also have antioxidant and free-radical-scavenging properties. A certain strain of *Bacillus coagulans,* for instance, has been demonstrated to possess such powers.[15] And when researchers genetically modified a strain of *Lactobacillus* to produce a free-radical-fighting substance, they discovered that they could generate a colony that can help restore balance between free-radical scavengers and the free-radical production in skin.[16] Put another way, these probiotic soldiers keep the peace by managing the harmony between free radicals (the rogues) and free-radical fighters (the rebels).

Good bugs on skin may also help build collagen, increase hydration, and improve the appearance of fine lines and wrinkles. In fact both *Streptococcus thermophilus* and *B. coagulans* can increase the production of ceramides in skin.[17] Ceramides are a vital component of skin: they protect against moisture loss and support the skin's matrix to keep it supple and firm. These molecules naturally decline with age, so having bacteria around to keep production up is a good thing for aging skin. *L. plantarum* has also been shown to help promote repairs to the skin barrier, making it a possible therapeutic for aging skin.[18]

Healthy skin exhibits a slightly acidic pH, in the range of 4.2 to 5.6—a level that inhibits pathogenic bacterial colonization. This acidic setting also helps maintain a moisture-rich environment and control enzyme activity. Translation: your skin stays supple, strong, and hydrated. But as we age, that pH begins to change. After you reach the age of seventy, your skin's pH level rises significantly, which stimulates certain enzyme activity that has the negative impact of breaking down proteins (think collagen). Probiotics, however, can lower pH back down to optimal levels by producing acidic molecules that in turn restore enzyme activity closer to what it is in younger, healthy skin so it functions—and looks—better.

I could go on and on about the science of topically applied probiotics. To say this field is exploding is an understatement. In chapter 8, I'll give you a cheat sheet of what to look for in topical products, based on all this research. For now, let's turn to the science behind oral probiotics.

BOOST YOUR GLOW WITH ORAL PROBIOTICS

The father of the modern probiotic movement was born more than 170 years ago. The Russian biologist Elie Mechnikov is credited with being the first to determine how *Lactobacillus* bacteria could be related to health.[19] Mechnikov is also considered the father of immunology: he predicted many aspects of current immunobiology and was the first to propose the idea that lactic-acid bacteria are beneficial to human health. Winner of the 1908 Nobel Prize in Physiology or Medicine for discovering white blood cells that can engulf and destroy harmful bacteria and particles (phagocytes), Mechnikov recognized a correlation between the longevity of Bulgarian peasants and their habit of consuming fermented milk products. In fact, he coined the word *probiotic* to describe beneficial bacteria.

Mechnikov, who believed that toxic bacteria in the gut caused aging and that lactic acid could prolong life, drank sour milk every day. His work inspired twentieth-century Japanese microbiologist Minoru Shirota to investigate a causal relationship between bacteria and good intestinal health. Dr. Shirota's studies eventually led to the marketing of fermented products (probiotics) worldwide. I'll be encouraging you to consume probiotics by eating foods such as kimchi and yogurt and beverages such as kombucha, but it's also worthwhile to consider probiotics delivered via a capsule or pill.

The most studied star families of oral probiotics are *Lactobacillus* and *Bifidobacterium* (you'll note that these strains are found in many fermented foods and topical probiotics, too).[20] Several strains of *Lactobacillus* demonstrate widespread (systemic) anti-inflammatory effects.[21] *L. paracasei,* for example, has anti-inflammatory properties that help reduce the risk of many skin disorders from the inside out. It's been further shown to improve the skin barrier and prevent water loss (water retention is a good thing if you want glowing skin).[22] This strain is currently being studied for its effect on patients with rosacea, dry or sensitive skin, and atopic dermatitis (eczema). *Lactobacillus rhamnosus* GG ("GG" are the first letters in the surnames of Sherwood Gorbach and Barry Goldin, the scientists who isolated this strain of bacteria from a healthy human in 1983 and patented it) has been shown to help reduce the odds of eczema in babies at high risk for the condition whose mothers took the probiotic two to four weeks before giving birth as well as after delivery if they were breast-feeding—or if they weren't breast-feeding, when they added the bacteria to infant formula.[23] The prevalence of eczema in these babies was less than what's typically seen among babies at high risk for eczema whose mothers do not take probiotics. Another *Lactobacillus, L. plantarum,* may act as a potent antiager. In a 2014 study this strain reduced the number and depth of wrinkles in hairless mice compared to those in a control group.[24]

The *Lactobacillus* family can also reduce UV-induced sun damage in the skin. The results spoke for themselves when *Lactobacillus johnsonii* and 7.2 milligrams of carotenoids (the plant-derived antioxidant that gives vegetables such as carrots their color) were administered to healthy women for ten weeks before exposing them to either simulated or natural sunlight.[25] Compared to the placebo group, this dietary supplementation prevented the expected UV-induced decrease in Langerhans-cell density. Langerhans cells, you'll recall, are a critical part of your skin's immune system. They help inhibit unnecessary inflammation that can manifest itself in nasty, stubborn skin conditions. In this particular study, the scientists also concluded that the probiotic helped quicken the rebalancing of the participants' immune systems soon after exposure to harsh UV radiation.

The *Bifidobacterium* genus has a lot to offer, too. Several experiments on mice showed that the oral administration of *Bifidobacterium breve* prevented UV-induced damage to skin, which typically leads to a compromised barrier, water loss, and other adverse outcomes in the skin's health and functionality.[26] Translation: mice who ingested this healthy bacteria were less susceptible to damage from the sun. It was almost like they were drinking their sunscreen! Other studies have shown that *Bifidobacterium* can help lessen the production of free radicals in skin upon UV exposure.[27] Which means the bacteria can ultimately prevent the damage caused by those free radicals, including inflammation and accelerated aging in the form of more wrinkles and loss of suppleness as a result of less collagen production.

While I'm certainly not saying that a probiotic supplement is going to replace your sunscreen, you would do well to boost your skin's protection from the sun's harmful rays by both taking a probiotic and applying your sunscreen before you head outside. The more protection we have against UV rays, the lower our risk of skin cancer and premature signs of aging, such as wrinkles and brown spots.

Because of the prevalence of acne, studies that examine the effects of treating it with probiotics do continue to dominate, and once again we find that strains from the *Lactobacillus* and *Bifidobacterium* genera reign supreme. Small studies from Italy, Russia, and South Korea have shown that these bacteria also may help people better tolerate acne treatment in conjunction with oral antibiotics (yes, together, but spaced apart so the probiotic has a chance to work!).[28] A 2013 clinical trial demonstrated that oral antibiotics and probiotics might provide dual benefits, specifically for inflammatory acne.[29] When this study came out, I was not at all surprised. I prescribe probiotic supplements to all my female acne patients whenever I prescribe a course of oral antibiotics. Why? To prevent the well-known side effects of antibiotics, including stomach upset and yeast infections. Every so often, I'd have a patient return to me saying that, even though her oral course of antibiotics had ended, she had continued to take the probiotic supplement because she believed the supplement was helping her skin.

After hearing this story again and again, I started prescribing probiotics along with any antibiotic prescription I wrote, to both men and women (because it wasn't just yeast infections I was trying to avoid). The patients' acne cleared quickly *and* they experienced fewer side effects, just as the 2013 study confirmed. I realized that probiotics by themselves were affecting my patients' conditions for the better. That was years before this study came out.

Finally, I want to mention one other star player from a totally different strain: *Bacillus coagulans*. This gem has been shown to have positive effects on immune function to the extent that it may reduce the production of free radicals, which means it could potentially help control acne, though more studies are needed.[30] (There's a lot of data showing the relationship between free-radical formation and acne, so it would make sense that anything that inhibits free-radical formation would help prevent acne.)[31] This bacterium has a long history of being used to alleviate gastrointestinal problems such as diarrhea (including traveler's diarrhea), irritable bowel syndrome, and C. diff, which you know is my fave. It is also used to prevent respiratory infections (in fact a patented strain is advertised as doing just that by enhancing T-cell response to certain viral respiratory infections). We don't know yet exactly how this bacteria works to enhance immunity, but animal studies have shown that it may help regulate immune function and decrease harmful bacteria. Both these effects are good for skin health.

That's just the proverbial tip of the probiotic iceberg. I hope it's enough to get you excited about starting a probiotic supplement regimen today. Before you feel overwhelmed by all this information (and study after study) and try to take notes before running out to get your hands on a basket full of probiotics, don't worry: in part II, I will give you step-by-step instructions and guidance on what to buy, what to avoid, and how to implement a simple plan that will reprogram your microbiome from the inside out. What all this astonishing new information means, really, is that you get to control your skin health just by nourishing your microbiome. Even if you feel like you're at a disadvantage somehow (i.e., if you answered yes to a lot of the questions in the quiz on page 45), I have solutions that will help you turn the train around.

PART II

Glow with Your Gut

Welcome to the transformational phase in the process of cultivating a beautiful new you. Now that you've gotten a panoramic view of the gut-brain-skin connection, it's time to turn to the ways in which you can support the ideal health and function of your skin—from the inside out and the outside in. In this section of the book, we look in depth at the habits that foster a radiant appearance: diet, exercise, relaxation, stress reduction, and sleep. I will also cover skin-care rules and how to supercharge your skin with my "go-to-glow" supplement recommendations.

As you enter part II, feel free to go at your own pace as you implement my strategies and make lifestyle shifts. I will give you a detailed program in part III that is based on the information in part II, but I suspect many of you will begin to execute as soon as you learn. The faster you follow my recommendations, the sooner you will feel—and see—results. And remember, we're not just aiming for better skin. We're going to realize a whole lot more than that: increased energy, fewer chronic conditions such as gastrointestinal distress, reduced anxiety, better sleep, and a smaller waistline. All those benefits will lead to others, too, such as getting more done, feeling more accomplished, and simply enjoying life more.

Ready?

Set?

Let's glow . . .

CHAPTER 6

Feed Your Face

Dietary Recommendations for Putting Your Best Face Forward

The fact that the gut-brain-skin axis determines so much of how we look and feel from the inside out is accelerating our understanding of what it takes to have great skin. It's also revolutionizing treatments. The truth is that there is so much we can do starting today, just through diet. Solutions to chronic skin disorders are already at our fingertips. And it's so simple. This chapter focuses on my dietary recommendations and on explaining why, for example, it's important to eliminate certain commonly consumed foods from your plate. At the center of my message is the astonishing relationship between the food you eat and your body's and skin's biochemistry.[1]

Most of my patients lead super-busy lives and are often not thinking about what their lifestyle habits—especially dietary choices—are doing to their skin (perhaps this describes you). But you can't have great skin without a great diet, period. In addition to my in-office treatments, dietary modification is the most powerful tool for achieving the changes I want to see in my patients. It's also the most important area to address in terms of rebalancing the gut-brain-skin axis.

As you learned in part I, we delegate some of our bodily functions to the microbes that inhabit our bodies inside and out, and they out-number our human cells by a lot—possibly by as many as ten to one, though estimates do vary and scientists are still figuring this out. This new knowledge is both exciting and empowering because it means we are not bound by what we have inherited through our family histories or genes. We can change many things about ourselves that have a direct effect on our well-being and appearance, including the state of our microbiomes. We can adjust our food choices and dietary supplements; we can change how we take care of our skin, manage stress, and move our bodies; and we can even improve the quality of sleep we get. And all these things in turn can actually affect how our body's physiology behaves, right down to its genetic expression.

While we used to think that diet had little to do with the skin's appearance, we now know otherwise, thanks to new science, which I'll detail in this chapter. This area is one of my personal favorites, which is why I have devoted so much of my career to perfecting my knowledge of diet and the skin. There are countless simple food changes you can make to help your skin fight aging and build new collagen. For exam-ple, sprinkling just a pinch of cinnamon on your daily cappuccino or yogurt can improve circulation, giving you a healthy glow and trans-porting essential nutrients to the layers of the skin where collagen and elastic tissue are being produced. Leafy greens such as spinach and kale are an excellent source of zinc, which helps your skin break down old, damaged collagen, allowing new collagen to form.

You see, food is not just fuel. More than anything, food is informa-tion. It's data for your DNA and microbiome, sending signals to skin cells and its microbial communities and creating solutions to skin prob-lems. You must stop thinking that food is just a source of calories for energy or simply a source of micro- and macronutrients. Food actually talks to your cells and microbes—including those that thrive deep inside and the ones that coat your skin.

My dietary protocol will take you away from the typical inflammatory Western diet, which is high in unhealthful fats and sugars. It features fresh, whole foods (organic when possible) with an emphasis on low-glycemic ingredients. It allows for one serving of whole grains a day (e.g., one slice of sprouted bread or one serving of steel-cut oatmeal or quinoa) and limits refined carbs and dairy products (you can still eat yogurt, eggs, and certain cheeses). As you may know, low-glycemic foods will not raise your blood-sugar level—and insulin level—significantly. It's also important to note that all the recent scientific literature points to a strong connection between glycemic loads and risk for skin disorders.[2] High-GI (high-glycemic-index) foods trigger a cascade of endocrine responses that can cause skin issues by triggering the activity of certain androgens, growth hormones, and cell-signaling pathways.

You'll rejoice at not having to count calories or worry about portion control. Once you begin to eat in the manner I am prescribing, which allows you plenty of leeway to find the perfect diet for *you,* you'll rarely overeat again and should never get to the point of feeling so ravenous that you'll eat whatever's in front of you. This nutrition protocol will reprogram your body's sense of hunger and satiety so you'll be able to effortlessly eat the right amount of food for you—you'll know how much is enough based on genuine instinct. Now, that's an incredibly powerful place to be—a place where you no longer have a "diet mentality" and can trust your body's innate cues to tell you what, when, and how much to eat.

I should stress that everyone is unique in her own biological way. Because of this, not everyone can eat exactly the same things in the same quantities and look and feel great. The way your body responds to food is different from the way other people's bodies respond. Respect that fact and give yourself permission to experiment. This plan is highly customizable depending on your personal preferences. What I am offering is a basic template, albeit one that ensures optimal support of your gut-brain-skin axis. Modify it as you see fit. Keeping a food journal is a good way to identify patterns. Some people, for example, may be very sensitive to all carbohydrates while others might be sensitive to only high-GI foods, such as bagels and most breads, white potatoes, corn chips, doughnuts, and french fries. We'll cover all this in detail in the following pages.

Bear in mind that through dietary change, you are recalibrating not just your gut-brain-skin axis but also your taste buds and food preferences. In fact I think the biggest change you can make for the better when it comes to all this is to make an effort to alter your palate—slowly. I want you to go from craving sweets to appreciating tart, bitter, and sour flavors. Now, this won't happen overnight, especially since the food industry has helped us develop a sweet addiction, if you will, by adding sugars or artificial sweeteners to everything from salad dressings to protein bars falsely marketed as "healthy." But remember this: when you taste that sour flavor in those fermented foods rich in probiotics (e.g., sauerkraut, kombucha, organic Greek yogurt without any added sugar), you are feeding your gut what it needs to thrive. The first day or two is always a little rough, but soon enough you will wake up and the flavors you once craved will taste disgustingly sweet to you!

New science tells us that we can begin to change the health and function of our intestinal microbiome within a matter of *days*.[3] It is no wonder that rates of chronic disease rooted in the gut have gone up in tandem with rates of chronic skin disorders. The fact that the Western diet causes a slew of chronic diseases—from diabetes and heart disease to cancer and every manner of skin disorders—is no longer based on anecdotal evidence. Plenty of studies, some of which I've already covered, show without a doubt the destructive, inflammatory impact of the Western diet, which stresses quantity over quality.[4] Consequently we suffer from enormous nutritional voids.

What these studies demonstrate is that we are overfed and under-nourished. A diet high in sugar, processed vegetable fats, and synthetic chemicals and low in essential micronutrients and antioxidants is setting us up for the development of chronic inflammation—and as you know by now, our skin will show that inflammation in some way. Therefore the greatest form of medicine is to follow a dietary protocol that honors real, wholesome food that won't break your skin or harm its microbiome. Such a diet limits inflammatory foods, promotes nutrient density, and naturally supports the gut-brain-skin axis.

My dietary recommendations are rooted in years of working with patients and watching them transform themselves largely by following the same protocol laid out in this book. I've also done my homework enough to know the science working behind it. We have enough evidence to determine the best starting template for a body whose ailments manifest themselves in stubborn skin disorders. Wonder drugs do exist—in our food kingdom—and they can help you reclaim control of your skin in unfathomable ways. Where are they, and how do they work? Let's go to my Bowe Glow Food Rules. In chapter 10, I'll help you create meal plans based on the recommendations given below.

BOWE GLOW FOOD RULES

Whenever I give talks—either to the medical community, a lay audience, or patients in the office—I outline five simple, highly practical dietary rules that are all backed by science. I will walk you through each one of them.

- Go low-GI, whole, and unprocessed
- Be choosy with dairy
- Load up on antioxidant-rich plants

- Favor omega-3 fatty acids over omega-6 fatty acids
- Eat your prebiotics and probiotics

Glow Rule #1: Go Low-GI, Whole, and Unprocessed

Studies conducted on non-Western populations with a very low incidence of skin conditions (and in some where skin disorders are virtually nonexistent) have documented a common theme: an absence of processed foods and refined carbohydrates (i.e., no high-glycemic-index foods).[5] They eat closer to nature, as our hunter-gatherer ancestors did tens of thousands of years ago: a diet rich in healthful fats and proteins in which most of the carbohydrates come from low-GI fruits and vegetables. Refined sugar is not on the menu. Foods don't come out of boxes with labels on them. Not only do these populations have glowing skin, they also don't suffer from obesity, hypertension, or malnutrition. And cardiac death and stroke are extremely rare.

According to my research and that of my colleagues, of all the potential dietary culprits in cases of bad skin, carbohydrates rank among the highest on the list, if not at number 1.[6] This is especially true when it comes to acne, which is probably the most studied skin disorder in the world because so many people in developed nations suffer from it, and the numbers continue to rise. As I wrote in a 2014 paper, our genes have not changed, but our rates of acne have—significantly.[7] The evidence to date points to a stunning correlation between refined carbohydrates and acne—which became the main message of that paper. Numerous studies show that when people prone to acne alter their diets to reduce their sugar intake and favor low-GI foods, they experience reduced numbers of acne lesions, reduced severity of acne breakouts, and reduced sebum production. There are multiple biological reasons to explain the connection, but one that stands out is the effect that refined sugars have on spiking blood sugar, which in turn can also increase hormones that stimulate oil production. These hormones can even change the composition of your skin's oil, making it more prone to acne formation. I would go so far as to say that refined carbs exacerbate most skin conditions.

Understanding acne is often the bellwether for understanding the etiology of other skin disorders. In other words, what's good for remedying acne is also good for resolving most other skin issues. And when it comes to editing out the bad carbohydrates that will ruin your skin, nothing speaks louder than the glycemic index. It is the best "meter," or cheat sheet, for knowing what to eat and what not to eat.

Get to Know Your Glycemic Index

The GI was developed decades ago as a measure of how foods, particularly those containing carbohydrates, affect the amount of glucose in the blood. The GI uses a scale of 0 to 100 and ranks foods against the reference point of pure glucose, which has a GI of 100. Foods with a high GI—70 and above—are rapidly digested and absorbed, causing fast but transient (lasting an hour or two) elevations in blood sugar, which in turn trigger a spike in insulin, the hormone responsible for ushering glucose out of the bloodstream and into cells for use. Insulin also stimulates fat and amino acid uptake into cells and inhibits the body from breaking down stored fat, glycogen, and proteins. Typical high-GI foods are processed and filled with sugar and white flour. Low-GI foods—55 and less—such as leafy greens, quinoa, fiber-rich fruit, beans, lentils, and some starchy vegetables such as sweet potatoes and winter squash, are digested more slowly, producing gradual rises in blood sugar and insulin levels. Many of these foods, including asparagus and broccoli, hardly change blood sugar levels at all. Those foods that have a GI between 56 and 69 are considered "medium" and can be consumed in moderation. These include foods such as brown or basmati rice, and whole wheat breads and pastas (you can go to my website for a list of common foods and their GI ranking).

It's worth noting that some studies have demonstrated that the glycemic index is not absolutely fixed—our individual metabolic factors affect the way we process various foods.[8] In other words, a food with a GI of 50 might act like a 60 in me and a 40 in you, especially depending on how you combine that food with others. (Rarely do we eat foods in isolation.)★ Our bodies are different. While it's true that there's probably some variation, I still think the GI is, at a very basic level, a helpful tool for broadly categorizing foods by sugar load. What this also means, however, is that you need to be aware of how foods affect you. Only you can know. If a food that's low on the GI seems to give you trouble, avoid that in the future. Go by how you feel (and look) rather than what the chart says is good for you. Use your food journal to help document and uncover patterns and sensitivities you might not otherwise realize are there.

Using the glycemic index to choose the best foods will help you gravitate toward whole foods and steer clear of processed, packaged junk. On my protocol, you'll eliminate all refined carbs and flours. This includes all the crap that you know is not good for you: chips, cookies, pastries, baked desserts, candy, most commercial energy and protein bars, fried foods, and a lot of foods labeled "fat free" or "diet."

Sugar is in almost every packaged, processed food. It's quite unbelievable how ubiquitous it is today, but look for it and you will find it—

★ Sometimes you will come across the term Glycemic Load (GL) rather than Glycemic Index. The GL is another metric developed to factor in the carbohydrate content *per serving* because some foods that appear high on the GI actually do not contain enough carbohydrates per serving to raise blood sugar significantly. Watermelon is one such food. It has a high GI of 80, but its actual GL is low. The cheat sheet on my website simplifies this for you, and you won't have to memorize any numbers.

even in unlikely places such as hamburger buns, french fries, potato chips, and processed meats. It may be called something other than sugar—sucrose, fructose, agave nectar, high-fructose corn syrup (see page 122)—but sugar is sugar, no matter how you spell it. And it can be hard to avoid if you don't make a conscious effort. Also, be aware that the body handles fructose and glucose differently. Briefly, glucose— naturally occurring in many whole foods such as fruits and some vege- tables as well as whole-grain breads, pasta, and, to a lesser extent, legumes—can be converted directly into energy for cells to use. Your body recognizes it immediately, gets that insulin pumping to deal with it, then tells your brain to stop eating when it's had enough. On the other hand, fructose—a sugar found naturally in fruit and honey but also in refined and processed foods—goes directly to the liver to be pro cessed without causing an insulin release that helps control how much of it you eat. That's not a good thing. Because you don't get that insulin reaction, your satiety signals won't work, so it's easy to consume more fructose than is good for you. Moreover, fructose is more likely to get turned into fat in the liver than into fuel. The majority of the fructose we consume is not present in its natural form (i.e., as bound to glucose to make sucrose) or delivered in its natural source (i.e., whole fruit). The average American consumes 163 grams of refined sugars (652 calories) per day: of this, roughly 76 grams (302 calories) are from a highly pro- cessed form of fructose derived from high-fructose corn syrup.[9]

Fructose, especially the processed kind, is seven times more likely to result in sticky protein clumps called glycation end products, which cause inflammation (see page 32). Although it doesn't have an immedi- ate effect on blood sugar because the liver deals with it, large quantities of fructose from unnatural sources have long-term adverse effects. Numerous studies have shown that it's associated with impaired glu- cose tolerance, insulin resistance, and hypertension.[10] Moreover, it does not trigger the production of hormones key to regulating our metabolism, which is why diets high in fructose can lead to obesity and its accompanying metabolic consequences.

Sugar in any form causes multiple changes in our bodies, from our cellular membranes and our arteries to our hormones, immune systems, gut, and even microbiomes. Sugar is our modern scourge—we are not designed to tolerate the levels we consume today.

By Any Other Name

There are more than fifty names for sugar, among them:

Barley malt	Fruit juice
Beet sugar	High-fructose corn syrup
Cane juice crystals	Invert sugar
Caramel	Malt
Corn syrup	Maltodextrin
Crystalline fructose	Maltose
Date sugar	Rice syrup
Dextran	Sorghum syrup
Dextrose	Sucrose
Evaporated cane juice	
Fructose	

Sugars Classified as Artificial

Acesulfame potassium (Sunett, Sweet One)

Aspartame (NutraSweet, Equal)

Neotame (Newtame)

Saccharin (Sweet'N Low, Sweet Twin, Sugar Twin)

Sucralose (Splenda)

Remember from chapter 2 that many artificial sweeteners can damage your metabolism by actually altering the composition of your microbiome. They make you much more susceptible to overeating and can trigger spikes in insulin levels (increasing storage of fat). Food companies are now hiding these artificial sweeteners under obscure names in their products because of increasing public concern. The list of artificial sweeteners is long and continues to grow with new formulations. They not only lurk in many prepared foods such as salad dressings, baked goods, processed snack foods, "lite" and diet foods, and breakfast cereals, they can also be found in unexpected places such as toothpaste, liquid medicines, chewing gum, and frozen desserts.

Glycation-Related Aging

Glycation is the biochemical term for the bonding of sugar molecules to proteins, fats, and amino acids: the spontaneous reaction that causes the sugar molecule to attach itself is sometimes referred to as the Maillard reaction. Louis Camille Maillard first described this process in the early 1900s. Glycation also occurs when you brown the outsides of foods using high heat—for example, when you toast bread or fry a steak; it creates flavor and changes the color of the food. Although Maillard predicted that this reaction could have an important impact on medicine, medical scientists didn't turn to it until 1980, when they were trying to understand the relationship between diabetes and aging.

In biological systems, the Maillard reaction is a prominent feature of aging. In the late stages of the reaction, so-called advanced glycation end products (commonly shortened, appropriately, to AGEs) are formed. These harmful products are mostly created by nonenzymatic reactions between sugar and amino acids.[11] Consuming foods high in sugar and/or foods exposed to high-temperature cooking methods such as deep-frying, broiling, roasting, baking, and grilling can increase the total daily AGE intake by 25 percent compared to the average adult daily intake.[12] Research is currently under way to study the impact of low-AGE diets on inflammation and risk factors for conditions such as heart disease.[13] Consuming high-AGE foods speeds up the production of your body's AGEs and increases the level of circulating AGEs in the bloodstream.[14] Researchers have linked AGEs to hardened arteries, tangled nerves, wrinkles, and myriad disease processes. Collagen and elastin, the fibers that, as you know, keep skin firm and elastic, are among the most vulnerable proteins in this process.

To get a glimpse of AGEs in action, simply look at someone who is prematurely aging—a relatively young person with a lot of wrinkles, sagginess, discolored skin, and a loss of radiance. What you're seeing is the physical effect of proteins latching on to renegade sugars. No joke: scientists can document a parallel between how much sugar animals consume and how fast their skin ages.[15] More sugar equates with prematurely "old" skin that has lost its elasticity and suppleness.

Or check out a chain-smoker: yellowing of the skin is another hallmark of glycation. Smokers have fewer antioxidants in their skin than nonsmokers, and smoking itself increases oxidation in their bodies and skin. So they cannot combat the by-products of normal processes such as glycation because their bodies' antioxidant potential is severely weakened and, frankly, overpowered by the volume of oxidation. For most of us, smokers and nonsmokers, the external signs of glycation begin to show up in our midthirties, when we've experienced a certain amount of hormonal changes and environmental oxidative stress, including sun damage. But smokers will have more extreme signs of glycation.

Glycation, like inflammation and free-radical production, to some degree, is an inevitable fact of life. It's a product of our normal metabolism and is fundamental to the aging process. But we want to limit or slow down glycation, just as we want to control inflammation and free-radical production. And in fact glycation, inflammation, and free-radical production do share a relationship. When one of these biological reactions is in overdrive, it's likely that the other two are as well, at least to a degree. Many strategies to promote longevity and a youthful appearance are now focused on how to reduce glycation and even break those toxic bonds. But this cannot happen when we consume a high-carb diet, which speeds up the glycation process. Sugars in particular are rapid stimulators of glycation because they easily attach themselves to proteins in the body. And guess what: high-fructose syrup is among the top dietary sources of calories in America. This form of sugar increases the rate of glycation by a factor of ten!

When proteins become glycated, they become much less functional. They also tend to attach themselves to other similarly damaged proteins and form cross-linkages that further inhibit their ability to function. But perhaps far more important is that once a protein is glycated, it becomes the source of a dramatic increase in the production of free radicals. This leads to the destruction of tissues, the production of damaging fat, the breakdown of other proteins, and even changes in DNA. Again, glycation of proteins is a normal part of our metabolism. But when it's excessive, trouble lies around the corner. High levels of glycation have been associated not only with premature aging but also with kidney disease, diabetes, cognitive decline (including Alzheimer's disease), and vascular disease.

Keep in mind that any protein in the body is subject to becoming an AGE. Because of the significance of this process, medical researchers around the world are hard at work trying to develop various pharmaceutical ways to reduce AGE formation. But clearly the best way to keep AGEs from forming is to reduce your consumption of sugar in the first place, whether natural, processed, or artificial.

Glow Rule #2: Be Choosy with Dairy

After sugar, dairy products are probably the number two villain when it comes to skin disorders. But not all dairy: it appears that cow's milk, particularly skim milk, is a big offender for many people, and most of those people probably don't even know it. In multiple recent studies assessing the risk for acne among milk consumers, the data were clear: consuming milk and milk-based products (such as ice cream) can significantly ramp up one's risk for acne—sometimes as much as fourfold! Interestingly, these studies don't show the same results with yogurt and certain cheeses.

What's so bad about milk? Although the exact reasons behind milk's negative effect on skin health are not entirely known, what we do know is that two key ingredients are probably at play: the milk proteins whey and casein. Whey increases insulin levels, which can impede our ability to control blood sugar and our ability to reduce inflammation, and casein promotes the release of an insulinlike hormone called IGF-1 (insulinlike growth factor). In the body, IGF-1 works with growth hormones to reproduce and regenerate cells, which is a good thing. But if you have too much of it, it can work against you by fueling the biological cascades that lead to certain diseases, such as cancer, and skin disorders, such as acne. Casein has also been show to trigger immune responses in some people, which will of course raise systemic levels of inflammation.[16]

Both whey and casein have long been implicated in the development of acne.[17] Indeed, there is a reason behind why bodybuilders and athletes who consume whey-based supplements such as shakes and protein bars can suffer from severe acne. But as I've mentioned, it can affect even the casual consumer of protein bars, which is why you should look for bars and powders that are made with plant-based protein and contain less than four grams of sugar per serving.

Although conventional wisdom says that skim milk is better than whole milk, skim milk can actually be more problematic because it often contains higher levels of these proteins, which are added to make the milk taste less watery. The good news is that it is easier than ever to find alternative milks, many of which now come fortified with calcium and vitamin D. I recommend low-sugar almond milk to my patients who don't have nut allergies. Almond milk has a nice flavor and is naturally rich in minerals and vitamin E. For those who cannot drink (or don't like) almond milk, I recommend trying hemp, coconut, or flax milk.

Unfermented versus Fermented Dairy

The beneficial effect of probiotics on skin may explain why pasteurized, unfermented dairy products such as cow's milk are associated with acne but fermented dairy products, such as yogurt, kefir, and cottage cheese, are not. Remember that fermented dairy products contain naturally occurring beneficial bacteria; they are therefore a natural source of probiotics.

Unlike milk, yogurt (if it is free of added sugar) and cheese don't seem to have such negative effects. In fact the probiotics in yogurt can actually help boost skin health, for the reasons I've explained. Moreover, probiotics can calm inflammation. The fermentation process involved in creating probiotic-rich foods such as yogurt produces lower levels of IGF-1 than those you would find in milk. More research is needed to precisely understand why cheese can be good for your skin. Many cheeses do contain some probiotics and have less lactose than milk does. Although these factors make them a better choice for people who have trouble digesting lactose-containing dairy products, they don't give us any answers about why cheese is often not associated with skin disorders. That said, if you consistently break out or have more severe skin issues after you eat dairy-rich foods, you may want to try eliminating all dairy from your diet and see how your skin reacts. Note that you'll probably need to do this for a month or longer to really see if there is any impact on your skin.

> ### Top Cheeses for Naturally Occurring Probiotics
>
> Semihard cheeses: Monterey Jack, Colby
> Cheeses with holes: Swiss, Gouda
> Italian cheeses: Parmesan, Romano, provolone, mozzarella
> Specialty cheeses: Limburger, Muenster
> Mold-ripened cheeses: Brie, Camembert, blue cheese, Gorgonzola, Stilton
> Goat cheese
> Cottage cheese
> Sheep's milk cheese

Although eggs are often found in the dairy section, they are not technically dairy products. The word *dairy* refers to products that come from the mammary glands of mammals, which basically means milk and anything made from milk, such as butter, cheese, and yogurt. However, eggs are a phenomenal food, despite what you might have learned about the yolk and cholesterol when you were growing up. I disagree with diets that limit you to egg whites only. You may be cutting calories, but you are also cutting critical nutrients. That egg yolk is a nutritional pot of gold. Whole eggs are among the only foods that contain vitamins and minerals, antioxidants, and all the essential amino acids we need to survive. And they can have far-reaching positive effects on our physiology. Not only do eggs keep us feeling full and satisfied, they also help us control blood sugar, which, as you know by now, affects skin health. (And no, there has never been a study showing that eggs are linked to heart attacks!)

You'll see that I don't shy away from eggs in my dietary protocol. I often love to start the day with an egg scramble using leftover roasted veggies from the previous night. It sets the tone for blood sugar balance and gets me through a busy morning without hunger pangs. (Hard-boiled eggs are also great for snacks.) Because of the volume of sugar in popular breakfast foods—including many commercial cereals, muffins, scones, energy and protein bars, and granola—changing up just your breakfast alone can be powerful. There are so many things you can do with eggs, too. Whether you scramble them, poach them, boil them, or combine them with other ingredients, they're are among the most versatile foods in the world. Hard-boil a carton of eggs on a Sunday night, and you've got breakfast and/or snacks for the week.

Glow Rule #3: Load Up on Antioxidant-Rich Plants

Antioxidants are exactly what the word implies: free-radical fighters. They help squelch those damaging molecules, which foment a storm of aging processes and chronic disease (yes, skin disorders included). In 2015, a paper in the *Journal of Skin Cancer* delivered news that's now traveling fast in dermatology circles: antioxidants, especially those acquired through the diet, have been shown to prevent free-radical-mediated DNA damage and cancerous growths as a result of UV radiation.[18] Multiple laboratory studies have found that certain dietary antioxidants (e.g., vitamins A, C, and E) show significant promise in skin-cancer prevention. These results have also been substantiated by animal studies.[19]

The number of antioxidants added to skin-care products is growing. They are even being added to most topical skin-care preparations. Antioxidants found in grapeseed extract, green tea, pomegranates, apple extract, dark chocolate, and caffeine are joining familiar antioxidants such as vitamins C and E. When they work their magic, they can protect skin from the ravages of sunburn, inflammation, DNA damage, and skin cancers.

In chapter 8, I'll give you a list of antioxidants to look for in topical skin-care products; you'll also get some antioxidants by taking a multivitamin (see recommendations on page 186). But there's no better way to get your dose of antioxidants than through the foods you eat. You can do so primarily by incorporating colorful whole fruits and vegetables into your diet, but you can also find powerful antioxidants in other foods such as fish and in drinks such as green tea and coffee (coffee is some people's primary source of antioxidants!).

Most studies that evaluate the role of antioxidants in skin health show that dietary sources of antioxidants are more effective than supplements. High antioxidant levels—and the presence of carotenoids in human skin—can only be achieved through nutrition. Carotenoids consist of a family of pigments that are manufactured by photosynthetic organisms (i.e., plants) and some nonphotosynthetic microorganisms, but not by animals. This means that the only way we can get these antioxidants is to ingest food from the plant kingdom.

In fact antioxidants are the reason why the produce department is filled with such bright colors, for it is the antioxidants that supply colorful pigments. For example, lycopene makes tomatoes and watermelon red, and beta-carotene gives carrots and sweet potatoes their orangey hue. I should add that beta-carotene, which is a precursor of vitamin A, has been proposed as a possible dietary remedy for skin conditions in people who are extra sensitive to light, as are many fair-skinned individuals.[20] Beta-carotene can help reduce the severity of photosensitivity reactions in those people and boost their ability to tolerate sunlight.

Antioxidants do much more than give plants color. These chemicals help counter environmental attacks from UV radiation, bad bugs, fungi, and more. Vitamin E, for example, is one of the most important antioxidants in the skin: it protects sebum from inflammatory damage. Human skin keeps a supply of many of these nutrients. But the skin's supply can become depleted as it fights off free radicals. This is why we all need to replenish our antioxidants by eating lots of vibrantly colored whole fruits and vegetables—with an emphasis on the veggies—throughout the day. I recommend limiting fruit (with the exception of avocados) intake to one or two servings a day because of its sugar content. But you are unlimited in the vegetable department.

The Antioxidant, Anti-Acne Connection

New evidence suggests that free radicals and oxidative stress play a role in the initiation of acne.[21] It is now documented that people with acne tend to have low levels of cellular antioxidants and numerous markers of oxidative damage. Historically we have been taught the following sequence of events in the development of acne: first, follicles become plugged, then bacteria sets in, and finally inflammation results. New studies, however, suggest that inflammation might actually *precede* these other events. In fact the release of inflammatory markers is one of the first things to occur in the development of acne. One theory is that free-radical damage to skin's natural oil, or sebum, appears to be the match that lights the inflammatory process. The reaction caused by those rogue free radicals is called lipid peroxidation, or sebum oxidation. Based on this knowledge, I recommend that my acne-prone patients in particular try to get lots of antioxidants in their diets and use a serum with antioxidants in it prior to applying sunscreen in the morning.

Following are my top five personal favorite antioxidants, with information on what foods and beverages contain them. In chapter 10, you'll learn how to incorporate them into your diet.

- Vitamin C, to help synthesize collagen and prevent and treat UV-induced damage—oranges, red bell peppers, kale, brussels sprouts, broccoli, strawberries, grapefruit, guava
- Lycopene, to help stabilize DNA structures in the nuclei of skin cells and promote smoother skin—mostly found in tomatoes,

but there are small amounts in guava, watermelon, and pink grapefruit

- Polyphenols, to help repair damaged skin and restore elasticity — these are the flavonoids and catechins (powerful antioxidants) found in green tea, dark chocolate, blackberries, cherries, guava, and apples
- Zinc, to help support antioxidant pathways — oysters, red meat, poultry, beans, nuts, whole grains
- Vitamin E, to help protect sebum from inflammatory damage — found in almonds, sunflower seeds, avocados, olives, and spinach

Glow Rule #4: Favor Omega-3 Fatty Acids over Omega-6 Fatty Acids

Admit it: at some point in your life, you bought food with the "fat-free" label on it. Perhaps you were trying to avoid fats altogether, thinking they were making you fat. Weight-loss companies, advertisers, grocery stores, food manufacturers, and popular books have long sold the idea that we should maintain a low-fat diet. Indeed, certain types of fat, such as commercially processed fats and oils (trans fats), are associated with adverse health outcomes. But not so for unmodified natural fats, whether from animals or plants.

We need dietary fat to survive. In fact fat is one of the most important elements in skin health. Each skin cell is surrounded by two layers of fat, which make up the cell's membranes. Known as the phospholipid bilayer, they incorporate dietary fats into their membranes and are key to the appearance of plump, healthy skin. Here's something else to consider: your skin's surface houses fat-friendly bacteria. These microbes consume the oil found naturally on your skin, leaving behind a thin antimicrobial layer of beauty-boosting fatty acids. When you don't incorporate enough fats in your diet, you starve these microbes, and they can't protect you. You also starve your skin of the super-moisturizing lipids that it needs to get the Bowe Glow. And when you wash your skin with certain products, you wash the protective oils away, making your skin more susceptible to infection.

There is a particular type of fat that should be favored over others, though: omega-3 fatty acids, which are polyunsaturated fats. These are the essential fatty acids that have celebrity status in the dietary world.[22] The two critical omega-3s are eicosapentaenoic acid (EPA) and docosahexaenoic acid (DHA), which are primarily found in fish. A third, alpha-linolenic acid (ALA), is found in nuts and seeds. We need these fatty acids to function, and their benefits—from helping reduce inflammation to promoting brain function, lowering bad blood fats, and, yes, helping skin's appearance by controlling oil (sebum) production—are well documented. Omega-3s also help delay the skin's aging process by nourishing those skin-cell membranes and keeping them fluid, thereby staving off wrinkles. In turn, this boosts hydration and prevents acne. The trouble is, most people don't get enough omega-3s. Instead they're loading up on too many proinflammatory omega-6s. Currently the general omega-6 to omega-3 intake ratio in America is twenty to one. The ideal ratio is two to one.

Omega-3s can also counter the effects of processed vegetable oils in our American diet. Unfortunately, the typical Western diet is extremely high in processed omega-6 fats, which are found in many commercial vegetable oils, including safflower oil, corn oil, canola oil, sunflower oil, and soybean oil: vegetable oil represents the number one source of fat in the American diet. We do need some omega-6 fats in our diet, but the focus should be on those found naturally in many nuts, seeds, avocados, and eggs. Alongside omega-3s, omega-6s are part of the building blocks of healthy cell membranes and are important not only because they help produce the skin's natural oil barrier—critical in keeping skin hydrated and young looking—but also because they are essential to brain and immune-system functioning. If you don't get enough of these fats in your diet, your skin may be dry, inflamed, and prone to skin disorders (and you'll be a high-risk candidate for other serious health issues). Some studies show that people with psoriasis do better when they take essential fatty acid supplements in addition to their medication than when they take medication alone.[23]

The key is to avoid the abundant omega-6s that find their way into processed, packaged foods (think baked goods). You'll be doing that automatically on my protocol, bringing the ratio of omega-3s to omega-6s into better balance. You'll also be bringing other omegas, such as omega-9s, into your diet from natural sources, thus contributing to a healthful intake of fats.

Glow Rule #5: Eat Your Prebiotics and Probiotics

Throughout history, fermented foods and some beverages have provided probiotic bacteria in the human diet. For thousands of years, our ancestors exploited the fermentation process. Although for centuries civilizations didn't understand the mechanism behind the process, the health benefits of fermented foods and beverages were likely intuited. Long before probiotics became available as supplements from health-food stores, people have enjoyed one form of fermented products. Evidence suggests that food fermentation dates back more than seven thousand years, to wine making in the Middle East. People in China were fermenting cabbage six thousand years ago.

Kimchi, a popular and traditional Korean condiment, is considered the signature dish of the Korean peninsula. It's usually made from cabbage or cucumber, but there are countless varieties. Sauerkraut, another form of fermented cabbage, remains popular throughout central Europe. Fermented milk products, such as yogurt, have been consumed for thousands of years around the world.

Generally speaking, fermentation is the metabolic process of transforming carbohydrates (i.e., sugars) into either alcohols and carbon dioxide or organic acids. The chemical reaction requires the presence of yeast, bacteria, or both, and it occurs in conditions in which these organisms are deprived of oxygen. Fermentation was once described as "respiration without air" by the French chemist and microbiologist Louis Pasteur in the nineteenth century.

Lactic acid fermentation is a unique fermentation process by which foods become probiotic, or rich in beneficial bacteria. In this process, good bacteria convert the sugar molecules in food into lactic acid. In doing so, the bacteria naturally thrive and multiply. This lactic acid in turn protects the fermented food from being invaded by pathogenic bacteria: its acidic environment kills off harmful microorganisms. This is why lactic acid fermentation is also used to preserve foods. To make fermented foods today, certain strains of good bacteria, such as *Lactobacillus acidophilus,* are introduced to sugar-containing foods to kick-start the process. Yogurt, for example, is easily made by using a starter culture (strains of live active bacteria) and milk.

The ideal way to ingest a healthful, diverse array of beneficial bacteria is to obtain them from wholly natural sources, such as sauerkraut, yogurt, pickles, kimchi, and fermented drinks such as kefir and kombucha. My menu ideas (see page 217) will help you begin incorporating these foods into your diet. Friendly bacteria consumed in foods and beverages are exceptionally bioavailable (easily accepted by the body). They get right to work in helping you maintain the integrity of the gut lining, balance the body's pH, regulate immunity, and control inflammation. They also serve as natural antibiotics, antivirals, and even antifungals. In addition, probiotic bacteria suppress the growth and even invasion of potentially pathogenic bacteria by producing antimicrobial substances called bacteriocins. What's more, as these probiotic bacteria metabolize their sources of fuel from your diet, they help release various nutrients bound in the foods you eat so you can more easily absorb them. For example, they increase the availability of vitamins A, C, and

K as well as vitamins from the B-complex group. No doubt all these nutrients are part of the skin–health equation.

Food-borne *prebiotics* should also be part of your diet. Beneficial gut bacteria love to eat prebiotics, which fuel the growth and activity of your microbiome. You're already familiar with prebiotics if you know the importance of fiber in your diet. All prebiotics are a form of fiber that we cannot digest but that gets consumed by the beneficial bacteria in our gut to benefit us. (Note, however, that not all forms of fiber act as a prebiotic.) As our gut bacteria metabolize these otherwise nondigestible foods, they produce beneficial short-chain fatty acids and even help us meet our own energy needs (in fact 7 to 8 percent of a human's daily energy requirements are actually met by short-chain fatty acids).

Prebiotics occur naturally in a variety of foods, including chicory, garlic, onions, dandelion greens, collard greens, leeks, and jicama (see below). I'll show you how to build better prebiotic-rich meals using these ingredients. New studies are also emerging showing that prebiotics even have the ability to reduce glycation—the nasty process in which sugars bind to proteins and fats and have their way with the body, increasing free radicals, triggering inflammation, and compromising the integrity of the gut lining, not to mention skin health. Remember, glycation causes protein fibers such as collagen and elastin—the building blocks of healthy skin—to become stiff, discolored, and weak. This results in wrinkles and sagging.

Food Sources of Prebiotics

Raw chicory root	Raw onion
Raw dandelion greens	Cooked onion
Raw garlic	Raw asparagus
Raw leek	Raw banana

MORE TO KEEP IN MIND

If you eat according to the guidelines in this chapter and use my menu plan on page 217 to see how it all comes together, you'll be setting the stage for a balanced gut–brain–skin axis. And what will you be drinking? Whatever you like from the Beauty Bar.

The Beauty Bar

I used to be addicted to one particular brand of diet iced tea. I started with one a day, then I graduated to two or three a day, craving it the way some people crave coffee. I felt like I needed it! I also loved finishing off my night with a diet soda. I drank tons of water and even green tea, so I never really thought a few "diet" drinks throughout the day were doing any harm. But I always felt a bit of bloating and discomfort in my belly, and I would semi-panic at the thought of missing my iced-tea fix. I experienced that "Aaaaahhhhh" feeling when I took my first sip. Normal, right?

Then I went on a lecture tour in Sweden, and my busy schedule combined with the generally healthier culture there made it impossible for me to get my hands on anything "diet." I badly missed my iced tea during the first two days, but by the third day, I found myself getting into a new routine. Water and sparkling water started to satisfy my thirst, and by the end of the trip, I had completely come out the other side of withdrawal! My body didn't crave the fake sugar anymore. And I found that I was less bloated and irritable. I woke up with a flat tummy, and it stayed that way all day. I felt more in control and less like a diet-drinkaholic, desperately seeking my diet drink midday. When I got home, I promised myself I would never go back, and I've stuck to that promise to this day.

I encourage you to drink filtered still water, sparkling water, or kombucha tea, or try my detox water recipe (see page 236). Stay away from diet drinks and anything made with artificial sweeteners. Remember, artificial sweeteners change our gut bacteria in dangerous ways—increasing our risk for obesity, diabetes, and skin disorders. I can't tell you how many times I've fixed a patient's struggle with weight loss just by getting her to forgo artificial sugars.

If you drink coffee, have one to two cups in the morning, preferably black and organic, and then switch to tea. (Drinking regular coffee all day could affect your sleep.) If you drink alcohol, have a glass of red wine with dinner. Don't overdo alcohol—it is a well-documented skin villain because of its dehydrating and inflammatory effects, among others. But red wine does have its beauty merits when consumed in moderation, as it contains an antiaging, heart-healthy, anti-cancer antioxidant called resveratrol. Resveratrol stops glycation, the process of sugar molecules bombarding your cells. The slowing of this process aids in slowing the formation of wrinkles. White wine and rosé do not offer the same protection.

YOUR SKIN-FRIENDLY GROCERY LIST

Below is a cheat sheet of foods you can add to your grocery cart that support what we've covered in this chapter.

Dairy

- **Greek-style yogurt** contains probiotics, which keep skin clear and radiant (look for the words "live active cultures," and make sure the sugar content is low—less than ten grams per serving).
- If you like your yogurt extra thin, try **kefir**. Kefir is a fermented milk drink made from a mixture of beneficial bacteria and yeasts; it originated in the Caucasus Mountains, in and around Russia.

- If you prefer something that has a milder flavor than Greek-style yogurt, try **skyr** (pronounced "skeer"). Skyr is a Norwegian-Icelandic cultured dairy product that is commonly available.

- **Omega-3 eggs** are a bomb of nutrition. They are an excellent source of high-quality protein and omega-3 essential fatty acids. Look for omega-3-enriched eggs that come from cage-free chickens fed a diet of flax meal. And remember not to be afraid of the yolk. Egg yolks increase blood levels of HDL, the good cholesterol, and contain the B-complex vitamin choline and antiaging carotenoids such as lutein and zeaxanthin.

- Buy **almond or coconut milk** instead of cow's milk. These are great substitutes for regular milk because they contain skin-boosting nutrients and won't increase your risk for acne.

Fruit

- **Berries** are packed with wrinkle-fighting antioxidants and vitamins.

- **Bananas** are rich in vitamins A, B, and E, which work as anti-aging and skin-smoothing agents. But they are also among the fruits high in sugar, so don't overdo it (no more than one a day).

- **Oranges and grapefruit** are loaded with vitamin C, an antioxidant that slows down the signs of aging by helping your skin reconstruct collagen.

- **Apples** are unusually high in fiber. One whole medium-size apple with its skin can provide 25 percent of your daily fiber requirement, helping control your caloric intake and even feeding good gut bacteria. The fibrous pectin of an apple serves as a prebiotic.

- **Avocados** contain healthful fats that your cell membranes, including those of the skin, need to function, trapping moisture in and keeping toxins out.

- **Lemons, limes,** and their juices contain important phytonutrients that serve multiple health-promoting functions in the body, such as the stabilization of collagen and maintenance of elastin.

Vegetables

- **Dark leafy greens** such as spinach, chard, and kale are rich in carotenoids, which enhance immune response and protect skin cells against UV radiation and pollution. Their antioxidant, anti-inflammatory effects ultimately help block sunlight-induced inflammation in the skin. Leafy greens are also an excellent source of zinc, which helps your skin break down old, damaged collagen, allowing new collagen to form.

- **Asparagus** is not only a prebiotic (mostly when eaten raw), it's also one of the best sources of bioflavonoids, which strengthen small capillaries in the skin and may help prevent broken capillaries (which often show up in conditions like rosacea). It also contains an antioxidant called glutathione, which is produced naturally by the liver and is found within the cells. It plays a big role in a cell's ability to fight free-radical damage.

- **Tomatoes** contain lycopene, which becomes even more accessible to the body when the tomatoes are cooked. Ingestion of lycopene helps achieve smooth skin.

- **Squash and carrots** contain beta-carotene, a type of carotenoid and form of vitamin A that helps with skin-cell turnover, allowing dead cells on the surface to exfoliate and reveal healthy cells beneath. Note: drinking alcohol depletes the body of vitamin A, so after a night of one too many, power up with vitamin A–rich foods. Other good sources of vitamin A include **kale, mango, and watermelon.**

Fish

- **Trout, sardines, and branzino** (European sea bass) are loaded with omega-3s and protein. Studies have found that omega-3s help to combat inflammation of the skin, protect against sun damage, and achieve smooth-looking skin overall. Moreover, all three fish are very low in calories.

- **Salmon** (wild, not farmed) is rich in omega-3 fatty acids and is arguably the world's most heart-healthy source of protein. It also contains vitamins A, D, B, and E as well as calcium, zinc, magnesium, and iron, which all help keep skin young, supple, and radiant. I make salmon for my family at least twice a week. My daughter is convinced she is learning to read because salmon is "brain food"!

Animal and Plant Protein

- If you're a red-meat eater, indulge in **organic beef, bison, and game** once a week, but choose high-quality grass-fed meat. These will contain healthful fats and provide iron, which carries nutrients to skin, hair, and nails. You can eat white meats such as **chicken, pork, and turkey** more liberally throughout the week.
- **Legumes** include **beans, nuts, peas,** and **peanuts.** All are good sources of plant protein, fiber, zinc, and B vitamins.

Nuts and Seeds

- **Dry-roasted or raw unsalted almonds, walnuts, hazelnuts, and pistachios** are high in fiber, protein, and omega-3 fatty acids. **Macadamia nuts** are loaded with monounsaturated fats, and **cashews** are high in vitamin E (a powerful antioxidant). My faves are **pumpkin seeds** for zinc and **sunflower seeds** for vitamin E. As a bonus, the fat in nuts helps the body absorb nutrients from the produce you eat. I keep a plastic bag of nuts with me wherever I go, and I love mixing nuts and seeds into my yogurt to add a bit of crunch.
- **Chia seeds** are powerful antiagers containing omega-3 oils, antioxidants, and anti-inflammatory properties to keep skin and hair strong and healthy. They also qualify as a prebiotic because they contain soluble fiber that feeds intestinal flora.

Other Ingredients

- **Cinnamon** has been shown to boost collagen production. It also helps stabilize blood sugar because it increases cells' ability to use glucose by stimulating insulin receptors. What's more, cinnamon lowers cellular inflammation, which, as you know, is a prime age accelerator.

- **Old-fashioned (rolled) oats, quick-cooking oats, and steel-cut oatmeal** are high in fibers that enhance weight control, help stabilize blood sugar, fuel beneficial bacteria, and discourage cardiovascular disease.

- **Turmeric** has long been used in health and beauty circles. A natural anti-inflammatory, it contains active compounds—curcuminoids—that have many cell-protective properties and help even out skin tone and color. Turmeric, which is a member of the ginger family and is the ingredient that makes certain curries yellow, ultimately helps keep skin soft and supple while protecting against the oxidative stress that accelerates skin aging. I love to sprinkle it on my roasted veggies. (Note: turmeric does slow blood clotting, making it a factor in an increased risk for bruising. To minimize recovery time, avoid eating it before any medical procedure.)

- **Extra-virgin olive oil** is rich in a skin-smoothing emollient called oleic acid. The essential fatty acids in olive oil richly nourish the skin and have anti-inflammatory properties. Olive oil also contains polyphenols that act as potent antioxidants, some of which have been shown to improve general health and appearance and are rare in other consumables.

CHAPTER 7

Take Time to Recover

The Power of Exercise, Meditation, and Sleep

When forty-two-year-old Danielle came to see me about her out-of-control acne (which she'd never had as a teenager), rosacea, wrinkles, and brown spots, I instantly knew she was suffering from far more than just the side effects of aging, even if you took into account sun exposure, a poor diet, and lack of proper skin care. It was clear to me that Danielle was navigating stressful events in her life that were showing up on her face. She was even experiencing accelerated hair loss. "I see clumps in my brush and in my drain," she said. "People keep asking if I'm okay—I must look sick or tired all the time." When I asked her about how she handled stress or whether she took time for herself, she drew a complete blank. She wasn't expecting to hear that question from her dermatologist.

While it's common knowledge today that unyielding stress can be toxic to the body, people don't realize that many everyday habits can exacerbate that stress, which then changes the balance of the body's skin-friendly microbes in a negative way. Many of my patients, for example, have no idea how much their lack of exercise, troubled sleep, and technology addictions are affecting their skin, let alone their entire bodies. And when I prescribe such advice as "Get your heart rate up for twenty minutes daily," "Learn to meditate," and "Focus on your sleep habits," many people are surprised.

But it's true: if you don't take time to recover from life's daily stressors, you cannot have radiant, healthy skin. This goes deep down, all the way to the level of the microbiome. You learned a lot about the biology of stress and its effects on skin in chapter 3, and in this chapter we're going to explore the biology of rest and recovery in the quest to fix your skin. I'll make a stunning case for the power of three simple lifestyle interventions that can do more good than any cream, lotion, or dermatological procedure: physical exercise, meditation, and sleep. Scientists are finally unraveling the mystery behind the power of these activities in supporting not just the body's hormonal balance and underlying biological machinery but also its microbiome, which in turn helps support beautiful skin. The science behind these habits is truly breathtaking.

THE BEAUTY EFFECTS OF EXERCISE

We tend to think about the benefits of exercise in terms of fitness and weight control, but rarely do we consider its profound role in keeping skin looking young and firm. Surprising new research shows that exercise not only achieves this result but can also reverse skin aging in people who begin an exercise regimen late in life — proof that it's never too late to start! When a group of researchers at Ontario's McMaster University bred mice to age prematurely, regular exercise on running wheels was shown to prevent or even *undo* the signs of early aging.[1] These mice maintained healthy hearts, brains, reproductive organs, muscles, and fur (which didn't turn gray) far longer than their control counterparts, the mice forced to remain sedentary. These inactive couch-potato mice quickly grew frail, ill, demented, and graying or bald. The scientists theorized that if exercise could keep animals' skin from changing with age, it might do the same for ours. Lo and behold, further studies in humans showed that exercise—defined as at least three hours of moderate to vigorous physical activity a week—can indeed change the skin of old people so that it more closely resembles the composition of much younger skin. How much younger? In some cases, by as much as twenty years.

As you'll recall, the natural aging process of skin entails a gradual thickening of the outermost layer of the epidermis, the stratum corneum, which is made up of mostly dead skin cells and some collagen. But when we reach the age of around forty, it begins to change, getting denser, drier, and flakier. Meanwhile, the dermis layer, beneath the epidermis, begins to thin and lose elasticity; as a result, skin becomes translucent and looks saggy. These changes happen in addition to any others that occur from environmental damage. To think that we can slow down or even reverse some of these age-related changes through something as simple (and free) as exercise is truly astonishing.

While studies conducted thus far have used small sample sizes, the results demonstrated new findings about the benefits of exercise previously unknown in my field and have paved the way for more research. In 2015, the team of researchers at McMaster, led by Dr. Mark Tarnopolsky, professor of pediatrics and exercise science, revealed what could be happening when we break a sweat and raise our heart rates by looking at the effects of regular exercise on the skin.[2] Exercise affects the metabolism of the skin and the health of the mitochondria within skin cells. The mitochondria are tiny structures within certain cells that generate chemical energy in the form of ATP (adenosine triphosphate). They are unique in that they have their own DNA. It's believed they originated from ancient unicellular organisms that ultimately became part of our cells in order to produce a new source of chemical energy. Mitochondria are considered a third dimension of our microbiomes and have a special relationship with the gut microbiome. As we age, the health of our mitochondria degrades, thus impairing cellular metabolism. In effect, this is thought to cause age-related changes in skin—changes that can be thwarted or at least slowed down with exercise.

Tarnopolsky's team took skin samples from the buttocks (an area with limited sun exposure) of "habitually active" subjects who engaged in four or more hours of high-intensity aerobic exercise per week. They compared them to samples from sedentary subjects—people who exercised for an hour or less a week. Compared to their sedentary counterparts, the active subjects had significantly greater numbers of healthy mitochondria. As part of the same study, Tarnopolsky's team also conducted an intervention on a group of sedentary elderly individuals who underwent only twelve weeks of endurance training (via a cycling exercise program) and found that their healthy mitochondria levels increased. These changes were accompanied by improvements in the physical appearance of the skin. The researchers determined that the changes were dependent on post-exercise release of IL-15 (interleukin 15), which is a molecule involved in the immune response and is activated in response to viral pathogens.

The vascular aspect of exercise is also partly why it can be so good for skin health. When we begin to exert ourselves physically, there's an initial vasoconstriction of blood flow to the skin. But as we continue to exercise and our body temperature rises, vasodilation occurs, which means that our blood vessels dilate, or become wider. This increases the flow of blood to the skin. Over the long term, this causes positive changes to the vasculature that supports the skin. And with long-term exercise training, you can increase the peak amount of blood flow that travels to the skin—a good thing for skin's overall health and appearance.

I know that I'm not the first to tell you that, in addition to being good for your skin, exercise is an antidote for many things that can negatively affect your health. It improves every system, including metabolism, body tone and strength, and bone density. And, as you know, it helps you maintain an ideal weight. When you choose the right exercise for you, it's enjoyable, reduces stress while increasing your sense of well-being and self-worth, and brings you more energy.

Exercise Does a Body Good from the Inside Out

The following benefits of exercise have long been proved scientifically.[3] Note that many of these exercise-induced rewards correlate with reduced risk for skin disorders because of the skin's dependence on optimal metabolism, gut health, and hormone balance. Exercise also helps reduce levels of inflammation, which is one of the most powerful ways to prevent skin disorders.

Increased stamina, strength, flexibility, and coordination
Increased muscle tone and bone health
Increased blood and lymph circulation and oxygen supply to cells and
    tissues
More restful sleep
Stress reduction
Increased self-esteem and sense of well-being
Release of endorphins that act as natural mood lifters and pain relievers
Decreased food cravings
Lower blood-sugar levels
Weight control
Increased brain health, sharpened memory, and lower risk for dementia
Increased heart health and lower risk for cardiovascular disease
Decreased inflammation and risk for age-related disease, including
    cancer
Increased energy and productivity

Humans are designed to be active. But modern technology has afforded us the privilege of a mostly sedentary existence. Studies are now emerging, in fact, to show just how bad prolonged sitting can be.[4] It compromises metabolic health and increases the risk of premature death—regardless of age, body weight, or amount of physical activity! In other words, an hour-long session on an exercise machine will not necessarily undo all the damage caused by being on your butt the rest of the day (in front of the computer, driving, watching TV). This is why it's important to not only engage in physical exercise but also to get up and move throughout the day. You don't want to be sitting for hours on end, stagnating muscles and circulation.

Entire books can be—and are!—written about all the ways in which exercise boosts the body's physiology and, in turn, psychology. Bear in mind that multiple biological events take place in the body when we dance, take a cycling class, or go for a brisk walk. If you don't already follow an exercise program, this chapter will motivate you to start one as well as find ways to be more active throughout the day. And I promise to make this doable even for the most exercise-averse people. You do not have to train for a marathon or join a CrossFit gym. The simple truth is that you just need to find something you enjoy enough to want to do it regularly. Ideally, the chosen exercise will help you build and preserve lean muscle mass, flexibility, and what's called cardiorespiratory fitness. This means that your circulatory and respiratory systems are healthy enough to supply you with fuel and oxygen during sustained physical activity.

A comprehensive exercise program that lights up the body in healthful, beauty-boosting ways will therefore include cardiovascular work, strength training, and stretching. Each of these activities positively affects your metabolism and longevity and offers unique benefits that your body needs for peak performance. Plenty of activities fill the bill, from formal gym classes and classic sports such as swimming, biking, and running to at-home routines using streaming video over the Internet. Just be sure not to overdo it if you have not established an exercise routine already. Trying to do too much too fast will work against you, because you might burn out and become a couch potato again. Start small, maybe with thirty minutes of walking a day, and work your way up incrementally to a full and more comprehensive routine, perhaps with sixty minutes of moderate to vigorous exercise most days of the week and some weight training built into your routine two or three days a week.

For the most part, the benefits of exercise are cumulative. You can engage in short bursts of exercise throughout the day (which can help minimize the time spent sitting), or you can commit to a routine that blocks out an hour or so for your workouts on most days of the week. If you do dedicate a single period of time to your exercise regimen, do not allow yourself to be sedentary the rest of the day. I'll help you learn how to formulate a plan that works for you with the program outline in chapter 10.

OM-ING (SORT OF) YOUR WAY TO BETTER SKIN

If you are anything like I used to be, you are itching to skip this part, but *don't!* A few short years ago, if someone started talking to me about the benefits of yoga or meditation, I would immediately stop listening. I was a multitasker, a type A powerhouse. I was a sweater, a runner, a trampoline jumper, not a deep breather. Relax? That was just not in my vocabulary. But people who are crazy-efficient multitaskers actually need to read this section more than anybody else. I promise not to go crunchy-granola Zen on you. But here's why this part is so important: meditation is a shortcut to a calm mind—and, in turn, to calm skin. I try to meditate once daily.

Earlier in the book, I covered the mind-skin connection, a relationship that has led to the development of a field called psychodermatology, or psychocutaneous medicine. For our purposes, meditation has the goal of triggering what's called the relaxation response, a term popularized by Dr. Herbert Benson at Harvard Medical School. His goal was to describe what meditation achieves and to help spread the word about the scientific benefits of meditation in the Western world.[5] His seminal book, *The Relaxation Response,* was first published in 1975 and remains in print today. During the relaxation response, the body releases chemicals and brain signals that relieve tension in your muscles, slow down your organs, and increase blood flow to your brain. This response can reduce the pain, discomfort, and anxiety that often manifest themselves in skin conditions (among other things). Scientists now theorize that the biological events taking place during the relaxation response essentially prevent the body from translating psychological worry into physical inflammation. The experience of the relaxation response appears to change cellular connections in areas of the brain associated with reactions to stress. And the good news is that perfecting a daily practice that turns on your relaxation response can help you more easily cope with stressors in your life that persist or even worsen.

But traditional meditation is not the only way to achieve the relaxation response. In fact one of Dr. Benson's professional missions was to popularize other techniques for generating the same response—techniques that go far beyond the stereotypical chanting of om and lighting of candles. Yoga, progressive muscle relaxation, tai chi, repetitive prayer, focused breathing, visualization, and guided imagery are all practices that can trigger the relaxation response. One of the reasons why slow, deep breathing, for example, is so effective is that it triggers a parasympathetic nerve response rather than a sympathetic nerve response. When you perceive stress, the sympathetic nervous system springs into action, resulting in surges of the stress hormones cortisol and adrenaline. The parasympathetic nervous system, on the other hand, can activate the relaxation response. Deep breathing, whose effects you can feel in seconds, is the quickest means of flipping the switch from an agitated, high-stress state to a relaxed and collected one as your body calms down on many levels.

Among the studies to examine the effects of deep relaxation in general and meditation in particular was one that took place in 2005, when researchers at Massachusetts General Hospital published an imaging study showing how meditation promotes a relaxed state: the act induces a shift in brain activity from one area of the cortex to another.[6] The scans show brain waves in a stress center of the brain (the right frontal cortex) move to a calmer side (the left frontal cortex). Such a movement of brain activity to areas associated with relaxation may explain why meditators are calmer and more content after reaching a meditative state. Newer research tells us that meditation can turn on genes that are anti-inflammatory in nature.[7] And you already know that anything that reduces overall inflammation is good for skin health.

Remember, you can meditate — engage in an activity that triggers the relaxation response — simply by stopping for a moment to be fully present (mindful) with your breathing and controlling your inhalations and exhalations. Deep breathing can be done anywhere, anytime. If you've never meditated before, a deep-breathing practice twice daily will get you started and give you a foundation for working up to more advanced techniques. In the program, I'll be asking you to set aside a few minutes each day, preferably in the morning, to do some basic deep breathing. See page 152 for a deep-breathing exercise I like to use that is super easy to learn.

Basic Deep Breathing

Sit comfortably in a chair or on the floor. Close your eyes and make sure your body is relaxed, progressively releasing all the tension in your neck, arms, legs, and back. Inhale through your nose for as long as you can, feeling your abdomen rise as your stomach moves outward and your diaphragm contracts and moves downward. Sip in a little more air when you think you've taken in all the air you can. Slowly exhale to a count of twenty, pushing every breath of air from your lungs. Continue for at least five rounds of deep breaths.

Five Other Ways to Turn the Volume Down on Your Stress Levels

- Get out in nature (bike, hike, camp, go to the beach, or just walk outside)
- Summon feelings of gratitude by keeping a gratitude journal
- Be mindful of your social media use: set boundaries when it comes to checking e-mail and social media sites, and make a conscious effort to see and update your friends in person
- Don't watch TV or use a computer or cell phone when you sit down for a meal or engage with friends and family members
- Splurge on a spa treatment once a month or once every couple of months

---

BEAUTY SLEEP IS REAL

We don't call it beauty sleep for nothing. The body intuitively knows that sleep deprivation, especially when it's chronic, will do a number on one's appearance—more dark circles, more redness and inflammation, more fine lines and wrinkles, and an overall dehydrated complexion. (Sleep deprivation is now well documented as a factor in all manner of disease.) Sleep quality indeed affects skin function and health, and, surprisingly, your sleep and your microbiome have a lot in common.

The field of sleep medicine barely existed when I was in training, but today it's a well-respected area of study that continues to demonstrate that the amount and quality of sleep you get have an astonishing impact on every system in your body.[8] Sleep is not a state of inactivity or a zone in which your body momentarily presses the Pause button. It is a necessary phase of profound regeneration. Indeed, billions of molecular tasks at the cellular level go on during sleep to ensure that you can live another day.

From laboratory and clinical studies to entire books, much research has been devoted to sleep's sweeping role in our lives. Sufficient sleep keeps you creative, sharp, productive, and able to process information quickly. Your sleep affects how hungry you feel and how much you eat, how efficiently you metabolize your food, how strong your immune system is, how insightful you can be, how well you cope with stress, and how well you remember things. Sleeping for a longer or shorter time than what your body needs (for most people, this is between seven and nine hours in a twenty-four-hour period) has been shown to be associated with a spectrum of health challenges, from cardiovascular disease and diabetes to automobile and workplace accidents, learning and memory problems, weight gain, and, yes, skin disorders.

It helps to think of sleep as food and water for your skin. If you don't get enough of it, you deprive your skin of needed nourishment and hydration. Chronic sleep deprivation has a multitude of effects internally, mostly on our hormones, that result in visible consequences to the skin. Put simply, imbalances in the body will lead to imbalances in the skin. The body's cells regenerate during sleep, so when you don't get enough sleep, cellular turnover—including the skin's—comes to a halt, and you're left with a dull, compromised appearance. Moreover, sleep deprivation affects the skin's natural barrier function and can lead to dryness and increased sensitivity to irritation.

What makes sleep so important for your skin health has everything to do with its role in one particular biological phenomenon: circadian rhythms. We all have an internal biological clock defined by the pattern of recurring activities associated with the cycles of daylight and darkness. These are rhythms that cycle through repeatedly roughly every single day, and they include our sleep-wake cycle and the rise and fall of hormone levels and body temperature. When your rhythm is not synchronized properly with your body's expected day-night pattern, you won't feel like yourself. Something will seem "off." If you've traveled across time zones and experienced jet lag, or pulled an all-nighter, then you know—probably painfully well—what it means to have a disrupted circadian rhythm.

The thing to remember is that your circadian rhythm revolves around your sleep habits. In fact a healthy rhythm results in normal patterns of hormonal secretions, from those associated with stress and cellular recovery and renewal to hunger cues that tell you when to eat. Our chief appetite hormones, leptin and ghrelin, for example, orchestrate the stop and go of our eating patterns. Ghrelin tells us we need to eat, and leptin says we've had enough. Recent science that has put these digestive hormones in the spotlight is breathtaking: we now have data demonstrating that inadequate sleep creates an imbalance of both hormones, which in turn adversely affects hunger and appetite. In one well-cited study, when people were instructed to sleep four hours a night for two consecutive nights, they experienced a 24 percent increase in hunger and gravitated toward high-calorie treats, salty snacks, and starchy foods.[9] This is probably attributable to the body's search for a quick energy fix, which is all too easy to find in processed, refined carbs.

Cortisol should peak in the morning and wane throughout the day.

Levels of this stress- and immune-regulating hormone should be lowest after 11:00 p.m., when melatonin levels tend to go up. The pineal gland secretes melatonin, a potent antioxidant hormone that signals sleep: for millions of years it has alerted the human brain that it's dark outside, ultimately helping to regulate our circadian rhythm. Upon the release of melatonin, the body begins to slow down, lowering blood pressure and core body temperature, which helps induce sleepiness.

Now, here's where the latest research has gotten wild: there's a newfound connection between your microbiome and your circadian rhythm. An expanding body of research suggests that the friendly microbes in the gut may in fact be responsible for *regulating* our circadian rhythms. How so? Well, it turns out that our gut microbes have a routine, too. Like clockwork, they begin their day in one part of the intestinal lining but then move a few micrometers in other directions before returning to their original position. New research in mice shows that the regular timing of these small movements can influence our circadian rhythms by exposing gut tissue to a variety of microbes and their metabolites as the day goes by.[10] Disruption of this dance can affect us!

Two phases dominate sleep: the non–rapid eye movement (NREM) and rapid eye movement (REM) periods. NREM sleep in turn is divided into three stages, the first two of which are referred to as light sleep and the third of which brings us into slow-wave ("Delta") sleep — the most restorative kind. Finally we hit REM sleep — deep sleep — during which we dream. We progress from wakefulness to NREM sleep to REM sleep in repeated patterns throughout the night, with REM stages usually getting longer as the night goes by. A restful sleep will progress through four to six cycles of sleep without wakefulness between cycles, each cycle lasting between 80 and 110 minutes.

Multiple studies demonstrate that sleep informs inflammatory signaling and that lost sleep results in daytime inflammation, which in turn affects your immunity.[11] If you've ever noticed that you get sick more often when you're sleep-deprived, now you know why: sleep disruption can leave you more vulnerable to infection, among other problems. Chronic inflammation can also manifest itself in skin disorders. And you know what persistently high levels of cortisol will do: break down collagen. Not a good thing for your skin.

Now that you appreciate sleep's role in optimal functioning, which in turn factors into skin health, let's talk about how can you maximize your experience of sleep and free yourself from insomnia (a condition that 25 percent of Americans suffer from). I'll outline some advice below, and in chapter 10 you'll see how this fits into your custom program. In week 2, you'll be focusing on sleep habits. By then, you will have already made changes to your diet that will support restful sleep.

Stick to your number every single night. Everyone has different sleep needs. You probably know yours from experience. It doesn't take a technical sleep study to find out how many hours you need to feel refreshed upon waking and productive throughout the day without needing caffeine every few hours. Be strict about going to bed and getting up at the same time daily, 365 days a year. Despite what many people might believe, shifting your sleep habits on the weekends to catch up can sabotage a healthy circadian rhythm. It's better for you to capture that early night slow-wave sleep by making sure you're in bed before midnight.

Act like a kid at bedtime. Anyone who has kids knows that their prebedtime routine is ritualized. And for good reason: like Pavlovian conditioning, it prepares kids' minds and bodies for sleep. Similarly, you should set aside at least thirty minutes before bedtime so you can send cues to your body and tell it to get ready for sleep. Disconnect from stimulating activities (e.g., work, being on the computer, looking at your cell phone). Take a warm bath, listen to soothing music, or read. Do some deep-breathing exercises before lying down.

Limit blue light from electronics. Power gadgets down near bedtime or minimize blue light from screens by activating the "night shift" mode on tablets and smartphones. Most natural and artificial light contains a blue wavelength that interferes with melatonin production and stimulates the alert centers in the brain, keeping us awake. You may want to go the distance with this one and keep all electronic screens outside your bedroom. In 2015, neuroscientist Anne-Marie Chang and her colleagues showed that light-emitting devices impaired sleep and disrupted circadian rhythms.[12] Further, these effects extended beyond evening and into the following morning.

Keep it cool, dark, and clean. The ideal temperature for sleeping is between sixty and sixty-seven degrees Fahrenheit. Use a sleep mask or blackout shades (try a sound machine, too, if you like). Bedrooms should also be kept clean and tidy (clutter will stress you out!).

Mind other "sleep thieves." Drugs (including coffee and alcohol) do indeed affect sleep. It can take time for the body to process caffeine, so try to have a 2:00 p.m. cutoff time for caffeinated drinks if you have difficulty sleeping. Alcohol is a mixed bag with respect to sleep. While alcohol can make you feel sleepy, its effects on the body disrupt normal sleep cycles, particularly the restorative slow-wave sleep phase. Pharmaceuticals, whether over-the-counter or prescribed, can contain ingredients that affect sleep. For example, many headache remedies contain caffeine. Some cold remedies can have stimulating decongestants (e.g., pseudoephedrine, which is chemically related to adrenaline). Side effects of many commonly used drugs can also affect sleep. Be aware of what you are taking, and if they are necessary medicines, ask if you can take them earlier in the day, when they will have less of an effect upon your rest.

Reset your internal clock with early morning light. Satchidananda Panda, a professor in the Regulatory Biology Laboratory at the Salk Institute for Biological Studies, in La Jolla, California, has conducted a lot of research into the circadian clock, especially as it relates to our genes, microbiomes, eating patterns, risk for weight gain, and even immune systems.[13] One of his most important discoveries has been that light sensors in the eyes work in conjunction with the hypothalamus to keep our bodies on schedule. As you might recall, the hypothalamus is the part of the brain that links the nervous and endocrine systems and regulates many of the autonomic functions of our bodies, particularly metabolism. The suprachiasmatic nuclei in the hypothalamus receive input directly from the light sensors in our retinas, which then triggers certain genes related to our body's "clock." This is why exposure to early morning light helps reset our circadian rhythms. Getting out into the morning sun can help recalibrate your clock if you're not feeling refreshed from sleep or are chronically having trouble going to bed when you know you should.

Consider a sleep study. If you have tried all these approaches and still fail to get a good night's sleep, or if you find yourself relying on sleep aids for prolonged periods of time, you might want to consider undergoing a sleep study to rule out other issues, such as undiagnosed sleep apnea. Sleep apnea, which is very treatable, affects a whopping twenty-two million of us and is caused by a collapse of the airway during sleep: muscles in the back of the throat fail to keep the airway open. This results in frequent but brief cessations of breathing, which cause sleep to be fragmented. Dreamless sleep and loud snoring are telltale signs of sleep apnea. Of course, undergoing a sleep study will require that you spend the night in a sleep lab that can monitor and record your sleep. These centers are not as unusual as you might think. Many hospitals large and small offer these services.

The fact is that our bodies crave balance and regularity, from our sleep habits at night to our waking activities and patterns of eating and exercising during the day. When you exercise regularly, you trigger the relaxation response, and when you get a good night's sleep, you tip the beauty-balance scales in your favor. In the following pages, you'll learn more about how to schedule exercise, find time to meditate (or engage in another relaxation activity), and safeguard your sleep time.

CHAPTER 8

Handle with Care

Reassess Your Regimen and Commit Daily to Proper Skin Care

Nothing is more thrilling for me than helping people look and feel their best and using what modern medicine has to offer to achieve these goals, especially when it comes to having beautiful, healthy skin. In addition to my childhood experiences, which I shared at the beginning of this book, there were other factors influencing my decision to become a doctor. Initially I was attracted to the field of medicine because of my unusual household. My late father had been completely deaf since he was three years old. My mother, who has always been fascinated by the beauty of sign language, decided to enter a master's degree program at New York University that specializes in signing. Guess who lectured frequently at my mom's program? My spirited, charismatic father, who happened to be getting his PhD at NYU at the same time. That is where they met.

As a couple, they supported each other's dream to bring the conversation about disabilities into the mainstream and to show the world the value of the *person* behind a disability. My father became a disabilities rights leader, and my mom was first a teacher of the deaf and, later, a sign-language therapist for children with special needs. Our family friends were an eclectic and incredibly fun group of special-needs and mainstream kids and parents. It didn't take much effort for me to look past a disability to the person inside.

Fast-forward to today. My personal background fuels my unique perspective as a dermatologist. My ability to empower others through my work energizes and motivates me every day. Treatment can be transformative for my patients, not just physically, as their skin improves, but also emotionally, mentally, and even professionally—and I love it as much as they do.

In medical school, we students were able to spend what little free time we had shadowing experts in various fields so we could get a taste of what kind of medicine we might want to specialize in. As you can probably guess, I spent a lot of time in the dermatology department and was especially drawn to what was then called the acne clinic at the University of Pennsylvania. While shadowing a mentor in this clinic, I met people with severe acne. Some developed disfiguring scars from their lesions, and many more developed emotional scars: but as their skin cleared up, witnessing the evolution in their personalities and their growth in confidence had an impact on me. Teenagers who initially hid beneath baseball caps and endless layers of bangs, reluctant to make eye contact, would transform over the course of their treatments. They would come out of their shells, start dating, go out for sports teams or the school play, and perform better in their academic pursuits. I was moved and touched by these experiences; no other field offered anything like it. Then, marrying my love of microbiology and my immersion in scientific discoveries about the human microbiome, I became obsessed with studying the microbiome's influence on skin and applying that knowledge to my work.

The top two goals in treating your skin correctly should be to maintain its natural microbiome while giving it what it needs to stay healthy and youthful despite chronological and environmental aging. In chapter 4 you read about the science behind skin care as it relates to new developments about the microbiome. Here I'll give you my rules of the skin-care road, which will help you establish a routine (I'll present the specific daily morning and evening to-do lists in chapter 10 along with the program outline). The goal in this chapter is to give you a foundation for proper skin care, providing the information you need when you're searching for products or using at-home treatments. Included will be a conversation about proper exfoliation and experimenting with ingredients such as retinoids, which are famously known to remedy a slew of skin problems during every decade in adulthood. Because of the volume of information in this chapter, I recommend reading through it carefully before planning your new daily, weekly, and monthly regimens. Then use this chapter's information in tandem with the morning and evening protocol described in chapter 10.

One fact to keep in mind is that that each of our microbiomes is totally unique. They are like fingerprints—no two people have the same microbial communities. Although we are stuck with a certain genetic predisposition to skin disorders, our microbiomes are largely environmental. Their health and composition have a lot to do with our habits and our surroundings. It's like a twist on the classic nature-versus-nurture relationship: when it comes to our microbiomes, we have a chance to take control. We aren't doomed to develop whatever is programmed into our genes. Our microbial collaborators can influence our gene expression and, ultimately, our health. And one of the ways in which we take control is establishing the right skin-care routine, one that respects, honors, nourishes, and supports the body's microscopic friends. Shift your topical treatment goals from harassing or killing scores of bacteria to supporting the health of your skin.

A Note About Skin-Care Brands and Dermatological Procedures

It is beyond the scope of this book to go into detail about all the treatments available today, whether prescriptions, over-the-counter products, or procedures performed in a dermatologist's office. What's more, technologies change rapidly. By the time you read this book, a new drug or therapy could be on the market to address your skin issues. I recommend that you visit my website (www.DrWhitneyBowe.com) for the latest updates to my personal recommendations and thoughts about various products and procedures. I also keep a perennial list of my preferred brands on the site, under the heading "Dr. Whitney's Picks."

Make it a goal to see a dermatologist once a year to be checked for skin cancer and to talk about any conditions or concerns you may have that require a dermatologist's expertise. If you implement the strategies in this book in combination with dermatological help custom-tailored to your skin, the results will be phenomenal.

Many top industry leaders in both prescription-based pharmaceuticals and over-the-counter skin care have been pouring funds into R & D to find what skin-care ingredients are capable of shifting the balance of bacteria on the skin in a positive direction. This requires a lot of careful study and attention to detail. First of all, they have to think about how traditional skin-care ingredients affect the flora: which ingredients might kill off good bacteria, and which might promote the growth of healthy bacteria on the skin? The answer depends on what condition we are treating and where on the skin we are focusing (armpits, face, neck, back, hands, groin). Certain bacteria like to flourish in areas where we make oil (e.g., face, chest, back), whereas others like to settle into our folds and creases. This helps explain why people with certain skin conditions tend to harbor species in common. While research into skin-care ingredients that take the microbiome into consideration is still under way, there are lots of options on the market today, and the selection will only get better in the future.

Cleansing is no longer just about cleaning off makeup and dirt—cleansing products are now designed to take into account how their ingredients affect the skin flora. We are all redefining what "clean" means. American skin-care brands now understand that "clean" skin still has trillions of microbes creeping all over it. During my days in the microbiology research lab, I had to maintain the right temperature, humidity, and pH in order to encourage one strain of bacteria to grow while preventing another from contaminating my petri dish. I even had to put certain ingredients in the culture medium ("food" for the bacteria) that would selectively allow one strain to grow over another. That's where the research is now in the skin-care world.

As new science and its related products emerge, I will do the work for you. I'll look at the data and tell you which brands to buy and when to save your money.

RULES OF THE SKIN-CARE ROAD

Rule number one here is to know what your skin likes and doesn't like. Everyone is different, depending on her unique skin and the conditions she is trying to treat. If you are acne-prone and use benzoyl peroxide, for example, use it carefully and judge how your skin reacts to it. Benzoyl peroxide can deplete vitamin E from the skin, leaving it more vulnerable to inflammation. The chemical may also kill some of your good bacteria, so I'm a big fan of following any products containing benzoyl peroxide with an antioxidant serum, then layering a probiotic moisturizer on top of that.

I believe in encouraging a healthy balance in your skin every day through a proactive approach. Every time you do something to help your skin, it's an opportunity to shift that balance in your favor. There arc no shortcuts here. It's a daily commitment, like eating as many sources of probiotics as you can and scheduling time to relax or exercise. Sometimes you have to change your strategy based on the way your skin is behaving (it will change what it likes as you age in general and throughout the year). Your bacteria have a variety of needs depending on what time of year it is, how much you are traveling, what the weather is like, what kind of water you are exposing it to, and the messages and signals it's getting from within the body. You have to respond to those needs, and your response will vary—and should vary— throughout the year. Furthermore, no one size fits all. What works for your friend might not work for you. In other words, listen to your skin!

Remember to treat your face, neck, and chest as one "cosmetic unit." Most products we use on our faces should also be applied to the neck and chest, especially sunscreen, antioxidant serums, and masks. I can't tell you how many patients neglect their necks and chests and one day realize that these areas give away their ages.

A note about serums: antioxidant serums are important but often overlooked. They're a crucial supplement to the protection sunscreen offers from the free radicals contained in UV rays. Antioxidants are also key for fighting infrared damage and pollution. As you know by now, studies show that, like UV rays, infrared radiation can cause DNA damage and wrinkles. Indeed, the sun gives off half its energy in the form of infrared light! You can't see it, but you can *feel* it. Infrared exposure damages skin through heat. And it's not just coming from the sun. Infrared radiation can also be found in artificial heating devices such as cold-weather outdoor heating units, food warmers in kitchens, hot yoga studios, some hair dryers, and electric radiant heaters. These devices are also often found in industrial settings, especially where glass and paper are manufactured, where molten metal is used for welding, and where textiles are produced. Some glassblowers and professional bakers show signs of premature aging on their arms because of constant heat exposure!

As I'll suggest in chapter 10, you might want to have two types of serums—one for the morning and another for the evening. Each one will contain slightly different ingredients. There will be more UV-combating ingredients in the daytime serum and more retinol in your nighttime serum. Serums are not heavy and moisturizing, as your day-time moisturizer or nighttime face cream should be. Rather, serums are light, fast-absorbing, and packed with potent ingredients that provide your skin with lasting long-term benefits. Because they are not weighed down by the types of ingredients that make moisturizers and night creams so hydrating, serums are able to quickly and deeply penetrate your skin in order to deliver their high concentration of active ingredi-ents. They are the powerhouses of any skin-care line. While serums tend to be expensive because of their ingredients (especially if you buy them in upscale department stores), a little bit goes a long way, so this product will last you a good amount of time. Less expensive serums with high-quality ingredients are now finding their way into stores such as Target, Walgreens, and CVS. Don't judge a serum by its retail cover!

Rules for Sun Protection

In terms of topical regimens, using a sunscreen is the single most impor-tant thing you can do for your skin. The skin has an amazing capacity to renew itself—if you give it the right tools! The ingredients in sun-screen block out beauty-busting UV damage. And by blocking out environmental stressors, you're giving your skin a chance to renew itself. One 2016 study found that a single application of a broad-spectrum SPF 30 facial sunscreen daily for one year reversed UV damage on the face.[1] Specifically, study participants saw improvements of 52 percent in mottled pigmentation, 40 percent in skin texture, and 41 percent in skin clarity after a year.

One of the most common questions I'm asked in my office, on social media, and by my friends and family is which sunscreen I recommend. There are so many options on the market. I always say that the best sunscreen is the one you will actually use! It does not matter whether you prefer a lotion, spray, or stick. It matters that you use a broad-spectrum sunscreen every single day, ideally one that contains UV-blocking ingredients and UV-filter chemicals (more on this below). You can use a sunscreen powder or a sunscreen mist throughout the day to refresh the initial application. Use a mist if your skin is dry, a powder if it's oily. I also recommend wearing a lip balm with an SPF of 30 or higher. (Remember: you can always find up-to-date brand recommendations, based on the latest studies, on my website.)

When it comes to sunscreen, there are multiple factors that can make a product fail to protect your skin. Some tips:

• Make sure you're using enough for adequate coverage. As I always tell my patients, you need a shot glass full of sunscreen to properly cover your face and décolletage and other exposed areas, such as hands, arms, and legs.

• Apply it properly. This means putting it on fifteen minutes before you go in the sun. Reapply every two hours. For a typical day at work, I recommend applying once in the morning and possibly once at lunchtime if you plan to be outside (there are many new products designed to go over your makeup). Reapply after swimming. For a full day in the sun, reapply at least every two hours and after swimming or sweating. Use extra precaution near water, snow, and sand, because these substances reflect UV rays, increasing your chances of a sunburn. Also, always apply sunscreen when it's cloudy: 80 percent of the sun's rays penetrate through clouds.

• Use brands that pass quality assurance standards. Sometimes the packaging might not be entirely accurate. Although the Food and Drug Administration requires manufacturers to test their products, the agency doesn't do its own independent testing to verify claims. For this reason, I like to rely on studies conducted by Consumer Reports (www .ConsumerReports.org), which does lots of testing to verify that products work as advertised. There have been instances when a sunscreen supposed to be SPF 50 has tested as SPF 10.

• Don't use expired sunscreen. Check the date on your bottle! Also, if you left your sunscreen in a hot car or outside in the sun last year, throw it out. It won't work effectively anymore. Invest in your skin and buy a new bottle. Many of the best-rated options are very affordable.

• Think twice about "natural" or mineral sunscreens that contain titanium dioxide and/or zinc oxide but don't contain any chemicals that filter UV radiation. Yes, you can burn through these, and so can your children! I reserve these for patients who have sensitivities to chemical sunscreens, which is a much rarer problem than you might think. When people "break out" after using a sunscreen, it's almost never because of the active chemical ingredients. Ideally you want a sunscreen that has a combination of UV-combating ingredients.

Sunscreen use is so important that if you do nothing else to your skin, this one daily practice will save you from a lot of trouble with skin conditions, especially premature aging.

Rules for Exfoliation

In addition to regular sunscreen use, proper exfoliation is key to combating premature aging of the skin. Alpha hydroxy acids (AHAs, also called lactic or glycolic acids) and beta hydroxy acids (BHAs) are all-star performers when it comes to exfoliation. You can find these ingredients in lots of over-the-counter products, but they are also used in higher concentrations during chemical peels at the dermatologist's office. These formulations smooth skin's outer surface and speed up cellular turnover. They can also help fade brown spots, unclog pores, and smooth out fine lines over time, if used regularly. At the same time, however, they can make skin extra sensitive. If you use them too frequently, they can disrupt the skin barrier and consequently lead to inflammation that triggers skin conditions.

AHAs are water soluble and usually are derived from plant, fruit, and milk sugars. In general, AHAs are good for skin that is dry, dull, aged, uneven in tone, or damaged by the sun. BHAs, on the other hand, are oil soluble, which is why they excel at cleaning out clogged pores. BHAs, like salicylic acid, derive from man-made sources and are good for calming down redness and inflammation because they are chemically similar to aspirin (acetylsalicylic acid, or ASA). BHAs are the ideal option if you have acne, oily skin, blackheads, blemishes, and breakouts.

You can also exfoliate using products that do not contain chemicals and instead manually rub particles into the skin to slough away dead cells. Chemical exfoliation dissolves dead surface cells and debris; manual exfoliation scrubs them away. Both methods can be irritating depending on how abrasive those manual exfoliants are and how concentrated the chemical formulas are. Of course, how often you exfoliate also factors into the equation. The more frequently you exfoliate, the higher your risk for a reaction in the form of irritated, inflamed skin. On the day before you exfoliate, you do not want to use a retinol product. Avoiding retinol will help prepare the skin for exfoliation so it's not extra sensitive and vulnerable to irritation. Use of retinol and exfoliation together would be a double whammy that most people's skin cannot tolerate.

Exfoliation is a practice that takes some experimentation. Most people can get away with exfoliating their skin once or twice a week. Everyone will have her own tolerance for various methods and formulas. The key is to find that sweet spot where the exfoliation process is not igniting inflammation. On the one hand, you're getting rid of dead cells and stimulating new cellular growth to uncover that fresh, healthy glow. But you are also walking a fine line between polishing your skin to perfection and making yourself vulnerable to irritation. You can consider a visit to a dermatologist who can apply a chemical peel tailored to your unique skin needs. Just don't have your first chemical peel or even a facial on the same day you'll be walking the red carpet or giving a public speech. Start with a peel that has the lowest concentration of chemicals and work your way up to more intensive peels. Always give your skin time to heal from any irritation. If you have never exfoliated your face before, try a gentle product to start (avoid the word "intensive" on the label). Some of the strongest formulas contain mechanical *and* chemical exfoliants, sometimes a combination of non-abrasive microbeads or crystals and AHA or BHA. Fruit enzymes can also be part of the mix; these work similarly to chemical exfoliants and are gentler than scrubs. First timers should use a product that contains a single type of exfoliating ingredient (mechanical or chemical) and is designed for sensitive skin.

Warning: You Can Get Too Much of a Good Thing

AHAs and BHAs (page 168) and retinoids (page 174) can do amazing things for our skin. But I view them as special treats. They cannot be used liberally every day, especially if you use them together. If applied too frequently, or at concentrations that the skin isn't ready to tolerate, they can do damage. It's just like so much of everything else in life: moderation is key. Otherwise you risk an inevitable biological backlash!

Sugar Scrub Recipe

You can exfoliate your skin twice a week, but the way you exfoliate your face, neck, and chest should be much gentler than the way you exfoliate your body, especially those rough spots such as the elbows, knees, and soles of your feet. While a DIY sugar scrub is too harsh for most people's faces, I love this kind of scrub for the extra-thick areas of skin on your body. My favorite recipe is made with two ingredients: brown sugar and almond oil. Simply mix ½ cup of brown sugar with ½ cup of almond oil and apply it to those rough spots with your hands (remember: I strongly caution against harsh body loofahs, handheld scrubbers, and other tools intended to exfoliate). Rub gently in a circular motion for a minute or two. Then rinse and pat dry before moisturizing. Note that sugar is *not* okay in your diet, but it's perfectly fine to use as an exfoliating agent for your elbows, knees, and feet!

Rules for Topical Probiotics

Believe it or not, the first known mention of topical probiotics therapy occurred more than one hundred years ago. In 1912, initial research on "topical bacteriotherapy" using *Lactobacillus bulgaricus* to treat acne was suggested. It would be many more decades, however, before we'd understand how powerful probiotics can be when applied topically—and not just as an acne remedy but also as a remedy for a wide variety of skin disorders. In 2013, the American Academy of Dermatology named probiotics a "beauty breakthrough."

Probiotics are finding their way into myriad topical products today (by the time you read this, topical probiotics may even be called by a new name to differentiate them from the probiotics in food and drink). Research into how they can enhance skin health and its microbiome (and which particular strains of probiotics are the most beneficial to skin) is still under way, because the ways in which they interfere with the development of, say, acne and rosacea is very complex. But there are plenty of data thus far to make a case for putting probiotics in topical products, as detailed in chapter 5. To remind you, probiotics have repeatedly been shown to do the following when applied topically:

- act as a protective shield that strengthens the skin barrier;
- restore acidic skin pH, keeping bad bacteria at bay;
- maintain proper balance of the skin's community of microbes;
- alleviate inflammation and oxidative stress;
- lessen photoaging (light-induced damage from UV radiation);
- help keep skin hydrated and promote the production of collagen, fats, and ceramides.

Probiotics used in topical formulas can be derived from bacteria found in or on the human body—in the skin and gut—or in our environment, such as water and soil. We are learning now which source will be the most effective for the health of skin. Following are the four categories of probiotics-based topicals we are now seeing in skin-care products.

- Probiotics: live bacteria
- Prebiotics: food for the bacteria
- Postbiotics: purified small-chain fatty acids, small molecules, and metabolites made by the bacteria; also includes heat-killed bacteria, bacterial fragments, and lysed (broken up) bacteria

Claims you will see on products vary. Some are said to preserve or protect the microbiome and prevent skin conditions. Others are said to create shifts in the microbiome. The latter products are the ones designed to be used on unhealthy skin, to treat skin conditions, or to reverse the signs of aging.

So what probiotic strains should you be looking for? Here's a cheat sheet to help you find the best kind for your particular concerns. Check my website for updates as newer science emerges.

Strains shown to help with acne and rosacea:

Lactobacillus plantarum
Enterococcus faecalis SL–5
Streptococcus salivarius
Lactococcus sp. HY 449
Lactobacillus paracasei

Strains shown to help with sensitive and dry skin:

Streptococcus thermophilus
Bifidobacterium longum

Strains that may slow premature aging:

Bacillus coagulans
Lactobacilli strains (e.g., *L. plantarum*)
Streptococcus thermophilus

Some companies are formulating proprietary blends, and there's nothing wrong with that. Your topical probiotics may be used in combination with oral probiotics (see next chapter). Recall that some products will contain live cultures, whereas others will contain supernatants or extracts. Some formulations might even contain prebiotic ingredients, which encourage the growth of healthy strains by serving as "food" for the good bacteria already living on your skin. No one preparation has proved superior to the others as of yet. Efficacy has to do with the degree of scientific rigor each company uses to test its formulation.

My Honey Avocado Yogurt Mask

A yogurt mask not only delivers probiotics naturally, it also has exfoliating powers. Yogurt contains lactic acid, which, you'll recall, is a natural exfoliant. That and the soothing properties of the yogurt and its live active cultures are ideal for short-term exposure. Following is one of my favorite formulations; try it some evening right after your clean your face but before you apply your nighttime products. More recipes for face masks are on page 244; you'll be encouraged to try one during the program outlined in chapter 10.

Mash together half a peeled and pitted avocado and 2 teaspoons honey until the mixture has a pastelike consistency. Add one small container (6 ounces) plain Greek yogurt and mix until well combined. Spread a light coating over your face and leave it on for 10–20 minutes before rinsing off with warm water.

Rules for Retinoids

Along with basic sunscreen, retinoids are one of the most powerful, effective, and rigorously tested substances in all of dermatology. They have been around forever, and they work wonders. No matter what ingredients are trending, from caviar to snail slime to stem cells, we always seem to come back to retinoids because they truly deliver results. I recommend that my patients start using them when they're in their thirties, but if you haven't tried them yet and you're long past this age, don't panic. You can start now and still benefit from them. It can take patience and experimentation, however, to use a retinoid correctly.

Many people who first try them will experience side effects that lead them to think they are allergic to retinoids or can't tolerate them somehow. This is almost never true.

First let's define what a retinoid is. The word *retinoid* refers to a category of ingredients that are derived from vitamin A. Among the benefits of retinoids is that they stimulate skin-cell turnover so dead cells fall off and new ones rise to the surface. In other words, retinoids are a type of exfoliant, albeit stronger than AHAs and BHAs. A good retinoid will be more effective than AHAs or BHAs at helping exfoliate dark patches and evening out the texture of the skin so it feels nice and smooth. Also, retinoids help to stimulate collagen production, which is great for fine lines and wrinkles. They can even help smooth out the appearance of scars and stretch marks. And they are great for acne. Retinoids are so universal in the treatment of skin conditions that I love recommending them to patients who suffer from a variety of issues—they can get multiple benefits from a single source.

Retinoids come in both prescription and over-the-counter formulas. Retinol is the form you find in most over-the-counter products, but there are a number of generic and branded names for prescription products. Although you can find an over-the-counter retinol with a concentration as high as 2.5 percent, that is too strong for most first timers. Start with a lower concentration, say, 0.5 percent, and give your skin a few weeks to become acclimated to the retinol. Then you can try stronger formulas. Look for products packaged in tubes or jars that cannot admit air and light, which will degrade the formula. If you want to explore prescription-strength formulas, it helps to start with an OTC version first to acclimate your skin to the chemical so you won't suffer the side effects of a stronger version.

The biggest mistake people make when they first start using a retinoid is to apply it every night, which is far too often for most formulations on the market today. Within a week or two, this can lead to rip-roaring retinoid dermatitis—red scaly patches that usually start around the corners of the nose and trail down to the chin, accompanied by stinging and burning sensations. In those cases, the overuse of retinoid has compromised the skin barrier and led to an inflammatory reaction. When it comes to retinoids, it is all about finding that delicate balance. You want to gently push the skin but not overdo it.

Here's the key: start with an over-the-counter retinoid and apply it every third or fourth night. If you have super-sensitive skin, you might have to start with just once weekly. Although some retinoids are photo stable, meaning that they won't break down in daylight, most are recommended for nighttime use. As instructed in chapter 10, you'll apply it after you wash your face and before you apply your serum and moisturizer (unless your serum contains retinol, in which case you don't need a stand-alone retinol). After two or three weeks, see if your skin is doing okay. If you're not experiencing redness and your skin doesn't look or feel irritated (i.e., if there is no stinging or burning), then you can amp it up by applying the retinol more frequently. The goal is to increase your exposure over time without triggering those side effects, which themselves can end up doing long-term damage to the skin, both visibly and to its microbiome. Today there are so many topical options available to counteract the side effects of retinoids that almost anyone can tolerate their use. I have really sensitive skin, but I can either use a prescription-strength preparation once a week (Sunday nights are my retinoid nights), or a much milder over-the-counter version three times a week. Most over-the-counter retinol products come with built-in ingredients to help soothe and moisturize, helping mitigate side effects to the point where you may be able to use them every night. (Note: everyone will be different, and some people will not be able to tolerate daily use no matter how long they try to train their skin to do so.) Whether you're using an OTC or prescription-strength version, your daily serums and moisturizers will also help prevent serious side effects.

Retinoids are a "pangenerational" therapy. They can be used during each major decade of adult life, often for different reasons at each stage, because they confer multiple benefits. They can help clear acne in your twenties, control discoloration and dark pigmentation in your thirties, strengthen collagen and reduce fine lines and wrinkles in your forties, and help prevent precancerous changes in the skin in the fifties and beyond.

A Special Note About Generic Acne Products

Over time, an increasing number of branded topical prescription drugs have been replaced by generic alternatives. This is especially true when it comes to topical acne therapies. One of the most common topical acne therapies prescribed by dermatologists has been, and continues to be, a product containing two key ingredients: benzoyl peroxide and an antibiotic (such as clindamycin or erythromycin). When formulated by the manufacturer in a single product, the ingredients are usually well tolerated. Dermatologists will tell you that if you use topical antibiotics alone—not in combination with benzoyl peroxide—you will likely develop resistance to that antibiotic. In other words, it will stop working, and unhealthy multiresistant bacterial strains will proliferate on your skin. If the product also contains benzoyl peroxide, however, then the resistance is much less likely to occur.

But here's what happens in real life: the doctor writes the prescription (or nowadays, "e-prescribes" it through a computer that connects with the pharmacy) and then the patient learns at the pharmacy that it's much cheaper to buy the generic versions of the topical antibiotic and benzoyl peroxide separately. Here's the problem: generic benzoyl peroxide is notorious for irritating the skin. So once the patient experiences a reaction (e.g., red, stinging, flaking skin), she will stop using that tube and

---

keep using just the antibiotic. This is a setup for resistance and problems. You can avoid this situation by making sure you use a single product that contains both the benzoyl peroxide and the antibiotic. If your insurance won't cover that combination product, then ask for an acne prescription that is antibiotic-free. Some dermatologists avoid prescribing antibiotic-containing prescriptions altogether to skirt this issue, and there are plenty of incredibly effective antibiotic-free options available today.

Rules for Addressing Discoloration

I don't know any person who won't have, at some point, discoloration on her skin. Whether it's caused by the side effects of pregnancy hormones, sun exposure in the past, or a genetically acquired skin disorder, discoloration can be troublesome for millions of people. The most common type of discoloration I treat is hyperpigmentation, or dark spots. There are three basic categories of hyperpigmentation: melasma, lentigo, and postinflammatory hyperpigmentation. Melasma is characterized by dark brown or gray-brown patches of skin on the cheeks, forehead, nose, or chin. The two primary causes of melasma are sun exposure and hormonal shifts (such as those that occur during pregnancy). A lentigo is a pigmented flat spot that is darker than the surrounding skin and, unlike a freckle, does not fade away during the winter months. This type of hyperpigmentation may be caused by genetics and/or sun exposure. They are often called liver spots but have nothing to do with the liver! Postinflammatory hyperpigmentation (or PIH) is caused when inflammation occurs in the skin and leaves a stain after it resolves. For example, if you find yourself living with a brown mark that lasts for weeks or months after an acne blemish disappears, you struggle with PIH. Those marks are often much more distressing than the acne itself!

There are lots of skin-brightening products on the market today, many of which contain fruit enzymes to exfoliate dead skin and purge existing pigment. The most popular and effective ingredient is hydro-quinone. I advise using hydroquinone only under the supervision of a dermatologist. When you use a product that contains more than a certain percentage of hydroquinone, or use it for too long, it can, paradoxically, cause more pigmentation problems. So look for a hydroquinone-free formula that contains brighteners such as licorice, soy, marine extracts, kojic acid, or niacinamide and use it every day, applying it at night after you wash your face and before you apply anything else. Make sure to follow strict sun-protection guidelines while you're using these creams, because even a small amount of sun exposure can negate all the progress you are making with the brightening formulation and make it appear as though the spots are going nowhere. If you don't find that it works for you within eight to twelve weeks, see a dermatologist.

Rules for Buying into Trends

As I write this, a procedure called microneedling is making headlines. During microneedling (also called collagen induction therapy, or "the vampire facial" when combined with your own serum), a dermatologist uses tiny needles to create a microscopic tic-tac-toe board of controlled wounds to the skin. Your body reacts by naturally healing your skin and, in the process, building new collagen and elastin in the dermis. More collagen equals younger, firmer skin. It is ideal for tightening and lifting the skin as well as for minimizing acne scars, smoothing out pores, and countering the effects of photoaging, dull skin, poor texture, stretch marks, and body scars. It can help with fine lines and wrinkles, too; in fact a recent study showed that medical microneedling can increase epidermal thickness by a whopping 140 percent while also increasing and thickening collagen bundles in the dermis.[2] In addition, microneedling allows serums, topical gels, and creams to penetrate or infuse more deeply into your skin, rendering the products more effective. Up to 80 percent of a product can penetrate skin directly after microneedling, compared to a mere 7 percent with normal application on intact skin!

Okay, I sound like an advertisement for this procedure. But here is why I chose this as an example: inexpensive at-home microneedling devices have been marketed (brilliantly) lately. At this time, I don't recommend these so-called dermal rollers, because they are much less precise than the device I use in the office and can even create tears in the skin. Moreover, at-home dermal rolling can be very abrasive to your skin and can spread bad bacteria, leading to very serious skin conditions. My advice is: proceed with caution. Some at-home treatments are not interchangeable with the sophisticated equipment, impeccable results, and high safety standards of the procedures performed in a dermatologist's office. When a new product comes out promising amazing results (cue the Saturday morning infomercials), do your homework and ask questions. Don't be the first guinea pig. There's a lot you can do for your skin without buying into potentially harmful trends.

Rules Through the Decades

Entering a new decade in life is exciting. We often feel like we've reached a new milestone and anticipate that the ensuing years will bring novel adventures and unexpected rewards. A new decade can also bring its own set of challenges, especially for the body as it continues to age. This is not necessarily a bad thing, for aging is often a joyful, enriching experience—you gain more wisdom, more confidence, and more skills that make life easier to navigate. And many of us actually get *more* beautiful with age, even though we don't look twenty anymore! But your skin's needs will change, and to keep up with those shifting needs, you should adjust your beauty regimen accordingly. Let me give you some tips that will help you plan for your progression through the years. Indeed you *can* age gracefully.

Twenties: Sunscreen is key—every day, rain or shine. If you do nothing else during this decade, commit to daily sunscreen. Also, get used to using products containing antioxidants such as vitamins C and E. Both your sunscreen and antioxidants will provide protection against free radicals. Now is the time to protect and prevent. Consider adding glycolic acid and/or salicylic acid to your routine, either in the form of at-home products such as a presaturated pad that contains these ingredients (yes, they can be used together) or by undergoing in-office light chemical peels (no downtime, five-minute procedure). Remember, these ingredients exfoliate the skin, keeping it smooth and keeping pores unclogged. Just don't overdo exfoliation (see page 168). If you suffer from acne, you may want to start trying a retinoid.

Thirties: Add a retinoid to your skin-care routine if you haven't done so already. This is the decade when you'll start to see fine lines form and perhaps struggle with adult acne. This is also a great time to ask your dermatologist for laser treatments, such as microneedling (see page 179), that keep skin tight, lifted, smooth, and healthy. The doctor might also use resurfacing lasers and noninvasive tightening devices that employ ultrasound and radiofrequency waves. These devices will boost your collagen production, and the more collagen reserves you start off with, the better prepared you are for the future. It's like filling up your tank with premium gas before embarking on a long road trip! If you're proactive, you might start using botulinum toxins in your thirties to prevent facial lines from getting etched in over time.

Forties: Try amping up your retinoid use by either using it every night (if you don't already do so) or asking your dermatologist for a prescription-strength formula (if you don't already have one). Consider adding more topical antioxidants to your regimen, both in the morning and in the evening, by switching up your serum. Look for products containing peptides, growth factors, and other collagen-boosting ingredients to keep tipping the balance in favor of collagen production over collagen destruction. Give those cells the upper hand by feeding them with collagen-boosting ingredients from the outside in. Despite their best efforts with at-home skin care, though, many women begin to use dermatologist-administered fillers in their forties. Fat pads are falling down and in as a result of gravity, creating the dreaded "jowl"—loss of definition along the jawline. Eyes can look tired because fat pads start to pooch out. But using the right skin care at home, and combining it with a few procedures in your dermatologist's office throughout the year, can keep everything firm, tight, smooth, and lifted.

Fifties and beyond: This is the time to bring on heavier moisturizers and richer products in addition to collagen-boosting ingredients so that you can boost hydration levels in the skin (think ceramides, hyaluronic acid, coconut oil, and dimethicone). As we age, skin loses its ability to trap moisture, so it gets dehydrated much more easily than it did in decades past. Consider layering skin-care products—serum first and rich night cream on top—or even adding a few drops of oil to a night cream. This is the decade in which you should start rotating in the occasional hydrating mask and at-home devices to help your skin-care ingredients penetrate into the skin. There are incredibly hydrating sheet masks that take advantage of what we dermatologists call occlusion. These single-use cotton masks are presoaked with very hydrating serums. The mask creates an occlusive barrier, sealing in the active serums and helping push them into the skin. Additional at-home devices are emerging that also assist with product penetration. Adhesive patches, for example, embedded with painless, fast-dissolving microneedles loaded with antiaging ingredients, are being developed that will help deliver these ingredients into the deep levels of the skin, where they can be most effective. Nanotechnology and microspheres are other new technologies that formulators are using to enhance penetration of active ingredients. At-home devices taking advantage of various forms of heat energy and even micromassage therapy will also assist in the delivery of active ingredients into the skin. The biggest barrier to seeing results from skin-care products when you are over the age of fifty is simply that the products sit on the surface and never penetrate into the skin. When you pair the right technology with the right ingredients, that's when the magic can happen. This is an evolving field, one that holds incredible promise. And, of course, there are in-office treatments to consider as well.

TWO SNEAKY PERPETRATORS THAT LEAD TO BAD SKIN

Before we move on to supplement recommendations in the next chapter, let me give you two final tips about other skin-sabotaging villains most people don't think about that can ruin your efforts to bring out the very best in your skin: cell phones and medications.

Go hands-free. Use hand-free devices or earbuds when you use your cell phone. Not only do cell phones harbor bacteria (no, not the good kind I keep talking about!), they also trigger acne as a result of the friction of the phone against the face. And keep in mind that even just looking at your phone can lead to "necklace lines"—horizontal neck creases that form when you stare down at the screen. When using your mobile device, try not to look down, and keep a pair of headphones with you at all times so you're not constantly rubbing your dirty device up against your face.

Mind your medicines. Millions of people use pharmaceuticals to treat or remedy health conditions. But many drugs—be they oral or topical—may also cause skin-related side effects that your doctor (or pharmacist) won't mention. For example, some corticosteroids, headache medications, seizure drugs, and even some forms of birth control (the minipill and implants such as Norplant) can trigger acne. Some drugs, including combination birth-control pills (containing estrogen and progesterone) and even certain antibiotics and blood-pressure medications, can make your skin more sensitive to the sun and lead to sunburn or dark patches after sun exposure. Then there are drugs that lead to blisters, make your skin peel, make your hair fall out, and cause problems with your nails. Certain medications can give you hives, pus bumps, or even stain the white part of your eyes with dark spots. Even seemingly harmless topical OTC drugs such as your typical antibiotic ointments (Neosporin, bacitracin) and sunburn sprays (benzocaine) can cause red, itchy rashes called allergic contact dermatitis.

It would be too encyclopedic to list every medication that can cause a skin condition (and you would get very bored very quickly!). I bring this up so that you remember to be mindful of the drugs you take. Look at their labels and read about the potential side effects.[3] If you have skin conditions that are mentioned in the package insert (e.g., "may aggravate acne"), bring this up with your doctor and ask about alternatives that can treat your condition without affecting the skin.

CHAPTER 9

Supercharge Your Skin

Navigating the Supplements and Probiotics Aisle

For the most part, we can get all our nutrients, including vitamins, minerals, and probiotics, from our diets—and we should aim for that. Nutrients are best absorbed through real whole foods. But let's be honest: achieving optimal levels through diet alone *on a daily basis* is often not realistic today (at least not for me and my patients!). We are busy, and our dietary options can fall short once in a while, despite our best efforts. I do not want you to rely on supplements to meet your body's nutritional needs (and if you follow my dietary protocol, you won't have to), but you would do well to consider a few choice supplements in the name of skin health.

I've simplified my menu of supplements to make this easy. None of the items listed below will cost much, and they can all be obtained at your local pharmacy without a prescription. (Do, however, consult your doctor if you're already taking any medications or supplements; get the a-okay before adding new supplements.) Many grocery stores, especially large national chains, will also supply these. The ones I've chosen to highlight are the vitamins and supplements most helpful in accomplishing two important goals: first, supporting the gut-brain-skin axis by nourishing the intestinal microbiome, and second, giving the body what it needs to maintain healthy skin (and, I should add, healthy hair and nails). Many of these ingredients are contained in multivitamins, but not at levels I recommend. I do not want you to megadose on any of these (more does not necessarily mean better), so stick with my dosage instructions. You can, however, also choose to take a multivitamin if you wish—especially to get your trace minerals (more on this below). All these dosages are on the conservative side, so adding a multivitamin won't be harmful. I like to think of these supplements—with the exception of a daily probiotic, which I think everyone should take—as optional additions to your daily routine. Remember: it is always best to get the bulk of your vitamins through food, and if you follow my dietary protocol you'll be doing just that! Here are my go-to-glow supplement recommendations:

Vitamin E (400 IU daily): This fat-soluble vitamin is an antioxidant that stops the production of free radicals when fat undergoes oxidation. Current research is examining whether, by limiting free-radical production and possibly through other mechanisms, vitamin E might help prevent or delay the chronic diseases associated with free radicals, skin disorders among them.[1] In addition to its activities as an antioxidant, vitamin E is involved in immune function, cell signaling, regulation of gene expression, and possibly other metabolic processes. The term *vitamin E* actually is the collective name for a group of fat-soluble compounds with distinctive antioxidant properties. Vitamin E is very difficult to consume through diet because it's not found in many foods (sunflower seeds and some nuts contain this vitamin). Moreover, UV damage rapidly depletes vitamin E.

Vitamin C (1,000 milligrams daily): The vitamin famously linked with citrus fruits does a lot more than boost immunity. Vitamin C is also a powerful antioxidant that has beneficial effects on skin, which is why it's often added to topical products.[2] It not only promotes fibroblast proliferation (fibroblasts are the cells that produce collagen and other fibers), it also acts as an assistant (a "cofactor") in enzymatic activity that relates directly to skin health and function. It even controls some of the DNA repair that goes on in skin to forestall cancerous growths. Its association with cells that control skin pigmentation (melanocytes) makes it a helpful ingredient in products that address skin discoloration. Because this vitamin is so easily lost in our urine, it's ideal to consume vitamin C–rich foods throughout the day via fresh fruits and vegetables while also taking a supplement. Foods high in vitamin C include red peppers, kale, broccoli, brussels sprouts, tomatoes, and, of course, oranges (but please eat them whole—never juiced!).

Vitamin D (1,000 IU daily): Actually a hormone, not a vitamin, vitamin D is produced in the skin upon exposure to UV radiation from the sun. It participates in a wide variety of biological actions to promote health, including strengthening bones and increasing calcium levels. In fact there are receptors for vitamin D throughout the body, which speaks volumes about its importance. Both animal and laboratory studies show that vitamin D protects neurons from the damaging effects of free radicals and reduces inflammation—all good things in terms of skin health.[3] In 2017, a team of researchers at University Hospitals Cleveland Medical Center showed that oral supplementation of vitamin D can quickly reduce inflammation caused by a sunburn.[4] Vitamin D is also linked to the control of p53, a tumor suppressor protein. More specifically, p53 is a gene that contains the genetic codes (instructions) for manufacturing a protein that regulates the cell cycle and hence is important in reducing cancerous cells. We have evidence now that vitamin D deficiency and the development of melanoma—the most deadly type of skin cancer—are related. And here's another critical fact: vitamin D performs a lot of its tasks through its regulation of gut bacteria.

It is best to get this vitamin by consuming supplements (and foods and fortified drinks) rather than exposing oneself to skin-damaging sun. Foods such as salmon, mushrooms, cheese, eggs, and fortified products such as almond milk all contain vitamin D. The safe upper limit is 4,000 IU per day, so if you take a 1,000 IU supplement and eat a few eggs or a piece of salmon in a single twenty-four-hour period, you're still in a very safe range.

Should you get tested for a vitamin D deficiency? As of now, the jury is still out as to whether healthy people should get screened. According to US Preventive Services Task Force guidelines, evidence is insufficient to assess the risks versus the benefits of screening in people who have no symptoms of a true deficiency, including muscle weakness and bone pain. On the other hand, you should be tested if you have osteoporosis, if you don't absorb fat properly (for example, if you have celiac disease or have had weight-loss surgery), or if you take medication that interferes with vitamin D activity, such as certain seizure medications and steroids. So even though vitamin D testing is widely available, we don't have enough data showing that screening people who don't have symptoms or risk factors does any good!

Heliocare (up to three 240-milligram capsules daily): This supplement, known as a "sunscreen pill," contains a formula claiming to help protect one from UV light. It should not be viewed, however, as a replacement for topical sunscreen—it is a dietary supplement. Heliocare, manufactured at a pharmaceutical-grade facility, contains a patented specialized extract of *Polypodium leucotomos* (PLE), a tropical fern native to Central and South America that has been used for centuries as a remedy for skin-related conditions.[5] I've generally avoided mentioning brands in this book, but this is the one I do want to call out because other supplements containing this extract are not as well vetted and it would be best to avoid them. Studies have shown that the fern extract lengthens the time it takes for skin to burn when exposed to sunlight.

We don't really know exactly how it works, but our current understanding is that PLE acts as a potent antioxidant, protecting the skin from oxidative damage caused by sun exposure.

What I find especially attractive about this inside-out form of protection is that it can shield the skin from other sources of free radicals, such as infrared rays, blue light, and even pollution. While the best topical sunscreens are designed to filter out UV rays, they all fall short when it comes to protecting the skin against these other elements. Heliocare gives you one extra layer of protection against premature signs of aging and skin cancer. I recommend taking one pill every morning. If you're heading out into the sun, you can take it again thirty minutes beforehand, right before you apply your sunscreen. You can continue to take these supplements every two to three hours if you're staying out in the sun, up to a maximum of three capsules a day.

Calcium (500 milligrams daily): A common element in the human body, calcium is critical to the health not only of your bones and teeth but of all bodily organs, including the skin, where it plays a role in regulating the skin's many functions. Most calcium in the skin is found in the outermost layer, and if there's not enough there, your epidermis can appear fragile, thin, and dry. A lack of calcium in the skin will prevent the production of new skin growth and the shedding of dead skin cells. In other words, skin turnover comes to a screeching halt. Calcium ions also allow neurons to signal one another, which ties into the gut-brain-skin axis. It's fine to find a calcium supplement that contains vitamin D (in which case you don't need a vitamin D supplement).

Trace minerals: The minerals most essential to skin health are zinc, copper, and selenium. If you eat according to my dietary plan, you will not be deficient in these minerals. (Note: look for them in the supplements I've already recommended, to which they are often added. Alternatively, buy them separately at the dosages I suggest below or simply add a daily multivitamin that includes these trace minerals to your regimen, in which case you won't need to take them separately.) But I want you to be aware of how they factor into skin health.

- ○ Zinc (10–30 milligrams daily): This mineral works as an antioxidant, lessening the formation of damaging free radicals and protecting skin fats and fibroblasts. It also plays a role in helping heal and rejuvenate skin. Because zinc is involved with cellular turnover and immune function, it is thought to help reduce acne flare-ups. The amount you take will depend somewhat on your diet (zinc is naturally found in grass-fed meat, grains, oysters, sesame and pumpkin seeds, peas, and beans). For most people, supplementing with 10–15 milligrams per day is fine — especially if you have acne (see "Special Circumstances," page 196). You don't want to go overboard with zinc because too much of it will put you at risk for copper deficiency (large doses of zinc prevent the absorption of copper in the digestive tract). These two minerals work together. Do not take zinc on an empty stomach, for it can cause stomach upset and nausea. Aim to take zinc halfway through a meal or right after.

- ○ Copper (1.5–3 milligrams daily): This mineral gets added to lots of topical skin-care products designed to hide the appearance of wrinkles and maintain youthful skin. Copper peptides in these products promote the production of collagen and elastin, among other important skin structures, and act as an anti-inflammatory. Copper also benefits your skin when taken orally because it's a factor in many enzymatic activities that promote healthy skin, hair, and even eyes. (Copper aids in the production of melanin, which is responsible for eye, hair, and skin pigmentation.) Copper helps regenerate skin elasticity and repair skin damage. Good food sources of copper include dark leafy greens, legumes (especially beans), nuts and seeds, mush-rooms, shellfish (especially oysters), avocados, and whole grains.

○ Chelated selenium (45 micrograms daily): This trace mineral is an antioxidant that protects other antioxidants, such as vita-min E. Studies have shown that a deficiency in selenium may play a role in inflammatory skin conditions such as acne, eczema, and psoriasis. Selenium functions in an enzyme called glutathione peroxidase, which is important in preventing the inflammation that characterizes acne. Foods high in selenium include Brazil nuts, halibut, sardines, grass-fed beef, turkey, and chicken.

Before we venture down the probiotics aisle, let me say a few words about oral antibiotics. Many patients come to me with existing pre-scriptions for both oral and topical antibiotics from other doctors and ask me for refills (they will often show me a tube of topical antibiotic cream that's nearly empty and an empty prescription bottle that used to contain oral antibiotics). We dermatologists are not supposed to pre-scribe a topical and oral antibiotic at the same time for reasons you can probably guess by now: such a scenario fuels antibiotic-resistant strains of bacteria and contributes to the global antibiotics crisis. Oral antibi-otics prescribed for acne, for example, should only be taken for a maxi-mum of three months. They should not be used at the same time as a topical antibiotic cream. Then, after those three months, you are sup-posed to go on a maintenance regimen that includes a topical retinoid and no antibiotic. (If this describes you — you're using both oral and topical antibiotics — speak with your doctor about another strategy. I can't overemphasize how important this is! Your skin — and your microbiome — will thank you.)

Unfortunately, thousands of people around the world take oral antibiotics for years, which is a problem even when there's no topical antibiotic involved. This problem is compounded in countries where one can buy oral antibiotics over the counter. For patients with rosacea, many physicians will prescribe low-dose antibiotics for years, falsely thinking this is safe because the patients are on "anti-inflammatory" doses and not "antimicrobial" doses. However, we are now aware that even these low doses can disrupt the microbiome and affect overall health. (Antibiotics are also prescribed for psoriasis and eczema, but usually for shorter periods of time, when the patient is experiencing flares—e.g., a ten-day or two-week course of treatment. Even in these cases, it's better to help patients *prevent* flares by maintaining a healthy skin barrier than to *chase* the flares with antibiotics. Hence the huge potential for products that promote a healthy skin microbiome and a healthy skin barrier.)

If and when you do have to take an oral antibiotic, take your oral probiotic in between your antibiotic regimen. Do not take them together in the same swallow; if you take your oral antibiotic in the morning, for example, take your oral probiotic in the evening. This will help ensure that your probiotic has a chance to work without being interrupted by the homicidal power of the antibiotic! And if your doctor thinks it's okay to be on low-dose antibiotics indefinitely, find another doctor.

Probiotics (10–15 billion CFU each daily): While it's ideal to obtain your probiotics from fermented foods and beverages like kombucha, there's nothing wrong with taking a probiotic supplement. Overall, as you'll recall, probiotics control the development of the immune system, often shifting the immune response toward regulatory and anti-inflammatory conditions. This ability to modify chronic inflammatory states means that probiotics may have a role in treating chronic inflammatory conditions, ranging from inflammatory bowel disease to acne, rosacea, eczema, and premature aging resulting from the ravages of UV radiation. As you know, you can get probiotics by consuming foods such as yogurt with active cultures, sauerkraut, kimchi, and fermented drinks such as kefir and kombucha. However, it's worth noting that when you eat a container of yogurt, you can't really know how many "active cultures" you're getting. Live, active cultures are often quantified (and labeled) in terms of the number of CFUs (colony-forming units) per dose. The CFU is used to measure how many bacteria in probiotics are capable of dividing and forming colonies. It helps to think of a CFU as a single distinct bacterium. CFU labels are commonly found on probiotics supplements but are not regularly found on probiotic-rich foods and beverages. To ensure you're getting plenty of probiotics, consuming probiotic-rich foods and beverages as well as taking a supplement is optimal.

The probiotics industry is poised to explode. I am certain that, with time, we'll identify new species of helpful organisms that will make their way into various probiotic preparations that you can buy over the counter.

Remember: Probiotics Are Additions to Your Regimen

Please do not stop taking the pharmaceuticals that your doctor or dermatologist has prescribed for you. Probiotics do not replace drug regimens or sunscreen. They will work in tandem with any other protocol you are currently following. As a reminder, if you are taking oral antibiotics, schedule your probiotics so that you take them in the hours in between your doses of antibiotics.

To find the highest-quality probiotics, first go to a reputable store known for its natural-supplements selection. Ask to speak with the employee most familiar with that store's selection of probiotics, someone who can offer an unbiased opinion. Many of these stores have someone well versed in probiotics who works solely in that department. Probiotics are not regulated by the FDA, as pharmaceuticals are, so you don't want to end up with a brand whose claims don't match its actual performance. Prices can vary wildly, too. The salesperson can also help you navigate all the nomenclature, for some strains have multiple names. Most products (again, see my website for up-to-date brand recommendations) contain several strains, but some probiotics only have one. Remember, your gut contains *trillions* of bacteria, and each strain will have varying survival rates and health benefits. Various strains perform various functions, and until scientists decode all the connections (e.g., strain X is good for condition Y), you would do well to consume multiple strains, either by choosing a multistrain supplement or by combining two or more strains. This will ensure optimal results for your gut and skin. Everyone's gut is unique, which means what works for you may not work effectively for someone else. Your goal is to support variety in your gut community. The richer the rain forest—the greater the variety of gut bugs—the better for you and your skin.

Make sure your probiotic contains at least ten billion CFU per dose. Although you can buy probiotics that contain more than one hundred billion CFU per dose, you may want to start off on a lower amount and work your way up. Depending on the state of your gut, you may experience gas and bloating when acclimating to the probiotic and recolonizing your gut.

The technology used to package probiotics is changing rapidly. Companies want to be sure their probiotics not only have a long shelf life but also survive on their journey through the alimentary tract, so they get to the place where they can do some good! High-quality probiotics companies (again, see my website for specific recommendations) will provide some sort of assurance that their products remain viable until the expiration date and that they reach their target (the gut) without being harmed in the stomach by acids. Many use patented technology in their packaging process to ensure the viability and potency of their strains up until the day you open the package.

If your probiotic comes with a prebiotic, all the better. But if you're getting your prebiotics from your diet, then it's not necessary to make sure they are included in the supplement itself.

Ideally, find a mixture of species from both the *Lactobacillus* and *Bifidobacteria* genera, plus *Bacillus coagulans,* whose effectiveness in improving gut health and, in turn, immune and skin health is supported by a lot of scientific evidence. Here are my top recommendations. These species are very common in today's probiotics products and are easy to find:

Lactobacillus plantarum

Lactobacillus acidophilus

Lactobacillus rhamnosus

Lactobacillus paracasei

Bifidobacterium bifidum

Bifidobacterium breve

Bacillus coagulans

You'll sometimes see numbers and/or letters after the bacteria names on ingredients lists. For example, you might see something like "*L. acidophilus* DDS-1." These numbers and letters simply mean that the strain has been patented. For example, DDS-1 (in this case, "DDS" stands for "department of dairy science" at the University of Nebraska, which is where the bacterium was discovered) is a strain of acidophilus that has been isolated, characterized genetically, then officially registered with the US patent office. A patented strain of *Bacillus coagulans,* to cite another example, is called BC30. You don't necessarily need those numbers to make sure you have a high-quality product, but try to buy probiotics that have been verified by ConsumerLab, NSF International, or the US Pharmacopeial Convention (USP). These are reputable third-party organizations that have long histories of certifying wellness products. These organizations cannot guarantee that a product has therapeutic value, but their seal is a good indication that the product contains the amount of ingredients advertised on the label and that it is not contaminated with dangerous substances, such as lead.

Special Circumstances

- *For people who don't eat red meat, pork, poultry, or a lot of seafood:* I recommend a daily iron supplement of up to thirty milligrams daily. If you experience any side effects, such as upset stomach, nausea, or diarrhea, take the iron with a vitamin C supplement or citrus food to increase absorption. Alternatively, try a lower dose or look for an extended-release product.

- *For people who eat cold-water fish less than twice a week:* Supplement with one thousand milligrams daily of an omega-3 fatty acid that contains both docosahexaenoic acid (DHA) and eicosapentaenoic acid (EPA). There are documented concerns about omega-3-supplement quality, however, so look for one that is certified by the International Fish Oil Standards Program (IFOS). This will help ensure that you're buying and consuming the quantity of active ingredients stated on the label as well as avoiding contaminants such as mercury. Vegans and vegetarians should look for IFOS-certified fish oil derived from marine algae.

- *For people who have thinning hair and/or brittle nails:* Try adding a biotin supplement to your diet. Biotin is a B vitamin that may improve the keratin infrastructure—a basic protein that makes up hair, skin, and nails. Deficiencies are rare. The current recommended daily allowance for this supplement is thirty micrograms. You can supplement with thirty micrograms daily, then double to sixty micrograms daily after a month, then increase to one hundred micrograms daily after another month if the following foods aren't in your regular diet: eggs, nuts, beans, whole grains, bananas, cauliflower, and mushrooms. (Note: the safe upper limit is five thousand micrograms daily, so you're not going to overdose at one hundred micrograms per day. People at risk for low biotin levels include those on long-term antibiotic therapy, which, as you know now, is common in the treatment of acne and rosacea. Read your labels carefully. Micrograms [mcg] are not the same as milligrams [mg]. One hundred micrograms equals 0.1 milligrams. You don't want to megadose into the hundreds of milligrams. At very high doses, such as 300 milligrams, the supplement can interfere with certain lab tests—resulting in false positives or negatives. These include tests as diverse as ones for pregnancy and cancer. Tell your doctor if you take biotin supplements when any lab work is performed.)

PART III

Putting It All Together

Congratulations. You've gained a tremendous amount of information by this point in the book. You've learned more about how to take care of your skin than you probably anticipated when you started reading. If you haven't already begun to change a few things in your life based on what you've read, now is your chance. In this next and final part, you'll follow a three-week program, during which you'll shift your diet and rehabilitate your gut-brain-skin axis back to its optimal state of well-being. This will be the place where you feel—and look—as beautiful as possible.

Making lifestyle changes, even small ones, can seem overwhelming at first. You wonder how you can avoid your usual habits. Will you revert to your old ways? Feel deprived? Spend too much money on new products? And can you reach a point where following these guidelines is second nature?

This three-week program is the answer. It follows a simple, straightforward strategy that has the right balance of structure, affordability, and adaptability. It will honor your personal preferences and power of choice. It will equip you with the knowledge and inspiration to stay on a healthful path for the rest of your life. The closer you stick to my guidelines, the faster you will see results. Bear in mind that this program has many benefits beyond the obvious physical ones. Ending a chronic skin condition might be first and foremost on your mind, but the rewards don't end there. My hope is that you will see changes in other areas of your life. You will feel more confident and have more self-esteem. You'll be able to navigate stressful times with ease and feel more accomplished at work and at home. In short, you will be more productive and fulfilled. I know you can do this. The payoffs are huge.

CHAPTER 10

Three Weeks to Radiant

Your Plan of Action for Smooth, Youthful, Clear Skin

You are ready today. Don't procrastinate. Don't postpone. Don't wait until you "feel ready" or for a "better time." There is power in jumping in and getting started. You have that power right here, right now.

You are ready to take a new step forward in a direction that will transform your looks—and even your life—from the inside out. I predict that within a matter of days you'll have healthier skin. You'll also feel increased mental strength and calmness and clarity, which will allow you to be more resilient in the face of your daily stressors. You'll feel other chronic or recurring symptoms begin to ease, especially those related to your gut-brain-skin axis. And you'll likely watch unwanted weight fall off—without your having to really think about it and certainly without your having to suffer through hunger pangs. My ultimate hope for you is that you achieve your own unique version of the Bowe Glow. You will experience:

- radiant, healthy skin;
- sharper mental clarity, focus, and drive;

- reduced stress levels and accompanying manifestations of stress, including fewer skin symptoms, GI symptoms, and tension headaches;
- a newfound genuine confidence that stems from feeling and looking healthier;
- glowing from the outside in *and* the inside out as a result of more healthful eating and living;
- strength to start defining your own journey;
- attunement to your inner voice;
- eagerness to try new workouts, new recipes, new products, and new strategies;
- a release from feelings of guilt when it comes to taking time to recharge and decompress;
- renewed strength and dedication to your dreams; and
- the drive to step outside your comfort zone and discover "what if."

Over the course of the next three weeks, you will achieve three important goals:

1. You will establish a new way of nourishing your body and skin through dietary selections tailored to your needs. This entails catering to your microbiome—inside and out—in ways that help bring out the smoothest, clearest skin.

2. You will incorporate daily practices into your life that help reduce your stress and lower overall levels of inflammation (and, in turn, angry skin). This includes exercising, getting plenty of sleep, and using mindfulness tools such as meditation to find the focus that will enable you to lead your most healthful and productive lifestyle.

3. You will adopt a skin-care regimen that supports and maintains the optimal health and function of your skin and, as you now know, your mind and body.

Each week of this three-week program is devoted to one of these specific goals and is designed to help you establish a new rhythm and maintain these healthful habits for life. In the day or days before you press Go, use the time to get your kitchen organized, wean yourself from sugar as you clear out the boxed junk and replace it with real whole foods, and plan your upcoming week.

During week 1, "Focus on Your Gut," you'll start incorporating my dietary recommendations and using my menu plan, which you'll continue throughout the three weeks.

During week 2, "Focus on Your Brain," I'll encourage you to get moving physically, establish a daily meditative practice (or *some* practice that decompresses you), and ensure that you get at least seven hours of sleep nightly—weekends included.

In week 3, "Focus on Your Skin," you'll turn your attention to establishing a daily skin-care protocol that leads to glowing, healthy, happy skin.

I'll be helping you put all the elements of this program together and equipping you with strategies for permanently establishing these new behaviors in your life—because you *can*. Once you start to live these changes, they will motivate you to continue. Dive in. You will love the results!

PRE-GLOW PREP

Let's get all the tools you need in place so that you are ready to get glowing! First, pick a day to start and mark that on the calendar. Don't wait too long. Perhaps you begin *tomorrow*. Make the commitment. Then get ready.

Stock Up on Your Go-to-Glow Supplements

All the supplements I list below can be found at health-food stores, at most supermarkets and drugstores, and online. Some of my favorite brands can be found on my website (www.DrWhitneyBowe.com). Try to take your probiotics right before or after a meal. I also recommend taking other supplements with food for two reasons. First, fat-soluble vitamins such as vitamins A, D, E, and K are better absorbed if you take them with some fat. Second, some vitamins and minerals can cause nausea or heartburn if taken on an empty stomach. This is especially true of zinc.

In chapter 9, I suggested that you add a daily multivitamin as a source of trace minerals if you don't want to take individual zinc, copper, and selenium supplements. It's not the end of the world if you choose to take a daily multivitamin in lieu of some of these stand-alones. You are much better off taking a multivitamin than forgetting half your supplements because it's just too much of a burden to remember. If you take a multi in addition to some of these supplements, such as vitamins E, C, D, and calcium, you will not approach levels that are dangerous or come close to overdosing.

For more specific information about each of these supplements, refer back to chapter 9. And if you have any questions about dosages, perhaps because you have personal health challenges, ask your doctor to help you make the proper adjustments. The dosages listed here are generally ideal for most adults on a daily basis.

Vitamin E: 400 IU daily

Vitamin C: 1,000 mg daily

Vitamin D: 1,000 IU daily

Heliocare: Up to 3 capsules daily

Calcium: 500 mg daily

Zinc: 10–30 mg daily (with food)

Copper: 1.5–3 mg daily

Chelated selenium: 45 mcg daily

Probiotics: See page 192

Plan to start taking your supplements on the first day of your dietary protocol in week 1. Some people may want to add an iron and/or omega-3 supplement depending on their unique circumstances. Refer back to chapter 9 for those details.

WEEK 1: FOCUS ON YOUR GUT

When you think of healthful living and a healthy glow, do you also envision bright citrusy colors and a clean, crisp environment? I know I do! Let's make that happen to keep you motivated and focused. Your first order of business this week is to make over your pantry, which will be your ally in this process, and start preparing meals and snacks that will get your glow on. Below are lists of the swaps you'll make followed by additional tips and a full week's sample menu. I recommend that you read through all the information here in week 1, look at my sample menu, and decide how your meals and snacks will realistically work out this week given your personal schedule and commitments. Then organize your grocery shopping list to match. You're obviously not going to want to purchase everything listed in the "Replace" section all at once. You won't eat or use it all in a single week!

The most important thing to do this week is get rid of the foods that are sabotaging your skin (see the "Evict" section) and bring in the foods and drinks that will support you and your skin. While it may seem overwhelming to change your diet overnight, if you think about this in terms of baby steps, it won't seem so difficult. You're making little adjustments and substitutions. You're saying no to junk and yes to you and your skin! If you can't go cold turkey on, say, the diet soda that's been part of your life for as long as you can remember, reduce your intake incrementally. Wean yourself off it and be sure to have a great, Bowe-approved substitution that you love on hand. Your taste buds will respond quickly, and those cravings will wane. Make it a goal to be free of the items under the "Evict" category by the end of this week. I know you can do this!

Evict (this is a biggie, so take a deep breath before reading)

• All forms of processed and refined carbohydrates, sugars, and packaged foods, including chips, crackers, rice cakes, snack cakes, cookies, pastries, muffins, doughnuts, sugary snacks, candy, most commercial energy and protein bars, jams, jellies, preserves, ketchup and other condiments with added sugar, processed cheese spreads, fruit and vegetable juices, dried fruit, sports drinks, commercial bread and English muffins, soft drinks and soda (diet and regular), fried foods, refined sugar (white and brown), and corn syrup (I know, I know, but trust me, we have delicious alternatives coming your way)

• Artificial sweeteners, including those found in salad dressings, baked goods, processed snack foods, "lite" and diet foods, and breakfast cereals (for a list of common artificial sweeteners, see page 122). Don't forget the beverages that contain these chemicals, too. Get rid of those diet sodas and teas. No exceptions here. Just get it done. I had a tough time with this one, but I lived to tell the tale! And you can use small amounts of authentic sweeteners—see below...

• Dairy milk, ice cream

• Processed fats, including margarine, vegetable shortening, and certain vegetable oils (soybean, corn, cottonseed, canola, peanut, safflower, grapeseed, and sunflower)

Replace with (when possible and applicable, buy organic, wild, and grass-fed products)

• **Whole fruits and vegetables:** See chapter 6 for lists of these

- **Protein:** Fish (e.g., salmon, black cod, mackerel, trout, sardines, branzino, tuna), shellfish and mollusks (shrimp, crab, lobster, mussels, clams, oysters), poultry (chicken), fowl (turkey, duck), beef, game, pork, legumes (see chapter 6; these include lentils, peas, and beans)

- **Healthful fats:** Omega-3 eggs, extra-virgin olive oil, coconut oil, ghee, butter made from the milk of grass-fed cows, dark chocolate, avocados, avocado oil, avocado mayonnaise, seeds, nuts, nut butters (note: almonds and almond butter beat peanuts and peanut butter because they have a better omega-3 to omega-6 ratio as well as more vitamin E and iron)

- **Low-GI grains:** Whole-grain brown or wild rice (no refined white rice), quinoa, sprouted and multigrain bread, barley, oatmeal (traditional rolled oats, quick-cooking oats, and steel-cut oats)

- **Herbs, seasonings, spices, and condiments:** Fresh and/or dried herbs, spices, and seasonings will go a long way toward helping you add flavor to your meals. So will pure condiments such as mustard, prepared horseradish, balsamic vinegar, and salsa (i.e., those that contain no added sugar or processed commercial oils)

- **Healthful baking ingredients:** Almond flour, unsweetened cocoa powder, vanilla extract, pumpkin pie spice, cinnamon, cacao nibs, vanilla stevia drops

- **Real sweeteners:** Maple syrup, honey, stevia, coconut sugar, unrefined brown and white table sugar

- **Probiotic-rich foods:** Yogurt with live active cultures, kefir, sauerkraut, kimchi, pickles, soft aged cheeses such as Gouda and Swiss (note: while you can certainly become a pro at fermenting and preserving your own foods at home using the myriad recipes online, I recommend buying these from high-quality manufacturers to start. Improperly fermented foods could contain pathogenic bacteria that will make you sick)

- **Prebiotic-rich foods:** Chicory, garlic, asparagus, onions, dandelion greens, collard greens, leeks, jicama

- **Optional beverages:** Unsweetened nondairy milks (e.g., almond milk, coconut milk, flax milk, cashew milk, pistachio milk, pea milk, hemp milk), tea, kombucha, red wine

Watch out for foods marketed as "gluten-free." Many of these foods (but not all, of course) are just processed products—their gluten has been replaced by ingredients such as cornstarch, cornmeal, potato starch, rice starch, and tapioca starch. Just because a package says "gluten-free" does not necessarily mean that what's in it is a natural, wholesome food.

I want this first week to be as easy and fun for you as possible. So a great goal is to initially make all your meals yourself in your "new" kitchen so that you are in charge of your nutrition and your mission. We will get you going out to your favorite restaurants in no time. The key here is to start on your path and minimize distractions, temptations, and cravings while you are retraining your brain and body (and taste buds). By preparing foods yourself this first week, you also gain an advantage in that you will get the dietary protocol down pat. This will make all excursions outside your own kitchen easier—and more adventuresome.

You have probably already heard about the benefits of "shopping the perimeter" of a store. It's true: this is where the get-your-glow-on foods will be located. Those inner aisles are the dead zones—the places where the food sold in boxes, bags, and cans is found. They won't help you or your skin. Steer clear (unless you're looking for, say, extra-virgin olive oil or avocado mayo). If you buy anything that comes with a nutrition label on it (most fresh items such as produce, fish, and meats do not), become skilled at reading those labels carefully. Look for suspicious ingredients such as added sugar, partially hydrogenated oils (look for the words *partially hydrogenated, hydrogenated,* and *shortening*), and chemicals you don't recognize or can't pronounce. Shoot for less than thirty grams of total sugar consumption per day.

During week 1, focus on mastering your new eating habits. Starting on page 217, you'll find my delicious seven-day Bowe Glow menu plan, which will serve as a model for planning your meals. Like the rest of the Bowe Glow plan, it is customizable to your taste and lifestyle. The other good news about this dietary protocol is that it's incredibly self-regulating—you won't find yourself overeating or hunting for that candy bar at the bottom of your purse, and you'll enjoy feelings of total satisfaction for several hours before sensations of hunger hit you.

When you're strapped for time and don't have access to a full kitchen where you get to call the shots, prepare meals beforehand and pack them to go. Having precooked or prepared tasty foods at your fingertips is helpful. The same goes for super-convenient snacks such as pre-portioned packages of nuts and seeds. You can also visit my website for my favorite energy-mix recipes and travel-friendly foods. Fill a container with fresh salad greens (don't forget: you can get a boost of prebiotic power with dandelion greens) and add chopped colorful raw veggies and diced chicken or a hard-boiled omega-3 egg. Drizzle extra-virgin olive oil on top before eating. I actually carry little travel-size dressings that I make every Sunday night for the week, so I never get caught eating a dressing that is loaded with sugar or chemicals. I just measure one tablespoon of olive oil and two tablespoons of balsamic vinegar into each container, shake well, and stick each in its own Ziploc bag so it doesn't leak. And don't underestimate the power of leftovers! Many of the recipes in this book can be made over the weekend (and doubled) to cover multiple meals during the week. Think ahead when you plan your meals and make your grocery lists.

In the past decade, there's been a huge shift in the variety of food available at our markets. Unless you live in a remote rural area, you're likely to be able to purchase any kind of ingredient within a matter of minutes, whether that means visiting the organic aisle in your usual grocery store or venturing to a local farmer's market. Get to know your grocers: they can tell you what just came in and where your foods are coming from. Some additional tips appear below.

Try food journaling: You might find it helpful to keep a food journal throughout the program, especially this first week. I love using the MyFitnessPal app on my smartphone, but for those of you who don't want to bother with an app, simply writing down what you eat at each meal is useful. Make notes about recipes and ingredients you like, foods that seem to brighten your skin (e.g., when you eat wild salmon for dinner, your skin glows the next day), and foods you think might be giving you trouble (e.g., you feel bloated and break out when you eat carbs, even whole-grain carbs).

Go super-low-carb for one week: New studies show that short-term dietary interventions of several days can significantly alter the gut's microbiome. This means a diet very low in carbohydrates—one that nixes all breads and flours and allows carbs only from vegetables and low-sugar fruits such as avocados, bell peppers, tomatoes, zucchini, and pumpkin. You may want to try this and see if your skin improves. Then you can gradually bring back some low-GI carbohydrates such as oatmeal, quinoa, barley, and multigrain bread into your diet and see how you look and feel. If your skin flares or you experience other issues, then you know you may be super sensitive to these foods and need to be more restrictive of carbs altogether.

Look for bright and bountiful: The more colors on your plate, the better. Deeply colored fruits and veggies are key to making sure you're getting enough antioxidants in your diet (look for local produce with a bit of dirt on it at your grocery store or farmer's market).

Don't fear fat: Fat is not the enemy. Never feel guilty if you reach for healthful fats such as avocados, nuts, and nut butters. Just make sure the only ingredients are the nuts themselves and maybe a little sea salt (no added sugars in nut butters, please!). And remember, any nut or nut butter is better for you and your skin than peanuts and peanut butter.

Be flexible about timing: Don't fret over following old, obsolete, dumb rules about timing your meals. You don't have to eat within two hours of waking, for example, or eat every two to three hours thereafter. New science shows that there's metabolic merit to spacing meals further apart—letting the body experience a mini fast that revs everything up positively, from metabolism to thinking! If you follow my plan, you won't feel those blood-sugar lows every few hours and panic about finding your next meal. You'll be able to space your meals out more easily without cravings or fatigue. The only exception to this rule is that I recommend you try eating dinner at least two hours before bedtime. You can have dessert within thirty minutes of bedtime, but trying to sleep right after a large meal can affect your sleep cycles, and healthy sleep is critical to healthy skin.

Have a snack: It's fine to snack in between meals. Be sure to combine a little protein with healthful fat and fiber (see page 216 for ideas).

Don't drink liquid calories in your coffee: This is a big no-no. Ditch the mochaccinos and caramel lattes and learn to drink your coffee on the lean side, with small amounts of nondairy milk and stevia if necessary. You might as well eat an iced doughnut given how much sugar is hidden in most of these beverages!

Stick to pure oils: Ideally, cook with extra-virgin olive oil, avocado oil, coconut oil, butter made from the milk of grass-fed cows, or ghee (clarified butter). Coconut oil, avocado oil, and ghee work better than olive oil for recipes that use very high heat (at the smoke point, which is between 375 and 405 degrees). When you sauté vegetables, try using extra-virgin olive oil mixed with a little ghee. Avoid processed oils and cooking sprays, unless the spray is made from extra-virgin olive oil. (A note about coconut oil: there has been a lot of debate about coconut oil—some say it's good for you despite its high levels of saturated fat, while others tell a different story and caution against its consumption. Unfortunately, the research remains fuzzy. My perspective? It's fine to consume coconut oil in moderation, especially if you follow my protocol and do not consume a lot of carbohydrates in conjunction with it. Extra-virgin olive oil should be your staple, but there's nothing wrong with using coconut oil when a recipe calls for it or when you are cooking over high heat.)

Roast a batch of veggies twice a week: I roast a big batch of veggies every third night and keep them in my fridge. Then I toss them in my break-fast scrambles, add them to my salads at lunch, or eat them at dinner as a side dish. I call it my Bowe Glow veggie staple. It doesn't get any easier than cutting up broccoli, peppers (of all colors), asparagus, brussels sprouts, mushrooms, and onions and spreading them out on two large cooking sheets. Next I mince some garlic, mix it with olive oil, and pour it over the veggies. Then I roast at 350 degrees for about forty-five minutes, until the veggies are crispy on the outside. The garlic can be swapped for other spices (e.g., turmeric) depending on the day and your mood, and I sometimes sprinkle some dried basil or oregano or fresh rosemary sprigs on top of the veggies depending on what I'm craving.

What to Drink

Twice a week, make a pitcher of "detox water" by adding some detoxi-fying antioxidants to regular water in the form of lemon slices, mint leaves, blackberries, and cucumber slices (see my detox water recipe on page 236). Then start your day with a tall glass of this elixir. If you're short on time in the mornings or don't like drinking a glass of water upon getting out of bed, take this with you to the bathroom and sip it as you're getting ready for the day. I like to alternate between sipping my hot coffee and sipping a chilled glass of this water. It's my version of being a two-fisted drinker—I love the way the temperatures and fla-vors complement one another first thing in the morning.

Water is not the only drink on the menu. Have you heard of golden milk? Kombucha? Rooibos tea? I have some goodies in store for you (see the menu below for details!). Because hydration is so key for healthy skin, my mainstay is simply filtered water or my detox version. Hydration doesn't have to be boring! I've found that if you like it, you will drink it. But remember to stay away from those artificially sweetened low-cal "diet" drinks—not Bowe Glow approved! Below is a look at what your day in hydration might look like.

- Rise and Shine: If you drink coffee, have it in the morning, as I do, but don't load it down with sugar and dairy milk. Aim for no more than two cups of organic coffee per day, and take it black with a pinch of cinnamon if you can or add unsweetened almond milk. Tea is also fine as an alternative to coffee. I used to drink a mild blend of coffee mixed with a packet of Equal and a tablespoon of sugar-free hazelnut powdered creamer—the sweeter the better! After I learned about the effects of artificial sweeteners on the gut, I forced myself to drink my coffee black. Day 1 was just awful. But by day 2, I started to appreciate the bitter flavor and decided to embrace it. I experimented with dark, medium, and light roasts, and, for the first time since I started drinking coffee, I actually *tasted* the coffee! Then, a week later, when I added unsweetened almond milk and cinnamon to my cup of joe, I couldn't believe how much I appreciated the natural sweetness. I recently took a sip of coffee made the way I used to love it, and I had to spit it out! It tasted like chemicals and was disgustingly sweet—my body nearly rejected it.
- Midday Madness: If you want more caffeine later in the day, drink tea, preferably an antioxidant-rich green or oolong tea. At lunch or with an afternoon snack, get creative and go for a probiotic-rich kombucha tea. I drink one bottle of kombucha a day instead of a diet soda or diet iced tea. Fortunately, you can buy high-quality bottled

kombucha tea in most grocery stores, because this is not a drink you'll want to make on your own. When switching to caffeine-free teas, try an anti-inflammatory rooibos tea.

• Dinner Delight: Remember, you can have a glass of red wine with dinner. Make sure to drink water, too.

• Bedtime Prep: Before bed, I love a cup of chamomile or rooibos tea. When I have a few minutes to spare, I love to make a warm cup of Golden Milk (see page 235).

Snack Ideas

• A handful of raw nuts (my favorites for the skin are almonds, cashews, pecans, and walnuts)

• Julienned raw vegetables (e.g., celery, carrots, bell peppers, broccoli, cucumber, radishes) dipped in two tablespoons guacamole, tapenade, hummus, a nut butter, or Savory Avo-Yogurt Dip (see page 242)

• A protein bar made with plant-based protein and less than four grams of sugar

• A medium apple, sliced and dipped in one tablespoon almond butter

• A slice of sprouted-grain bread topped with smashed avocado, drizzled with olive oil, and sprinkled with a pinch of salt

• Four slices of cold roast turkey, roast beef, or chicken dipped in mustard

• One or two hard-boiled eggs

• A bowl of fresh berries and a few squares of dark chocolate (ideally, close to 70 percent cacao)

• Lactofermented vegetables such as pickled cauliflower, carrots, and red bell peppers with Golden Milk (see page 235)

• A serving of Greek-style yogurt with active live cultures topped with cacao nibs, flaxseed, or chopped nuts (and vanilla stevia drops to taste, if desired)

- A protein smoothie made with a single scoop of plant-based protein, unsweetened almond milk, half a banana, and ice

SAMPLE MENU FOR A WEEK

Here is what a weeklong approach to your Bowe Glow diet could look like. All dishes for which recipes are provided appear in boldface. Recipes and additional cooking notes begin on page 234. For snacks, choose from the list above.

MONDAY

- <u>Breakfast</u>: Two eggs, any style, with a side of sautéed veggies and a slice of sprouted-grain bread, half a smashed avocado, and a drizzle of extra-virgin olive oil
- <u>Lunch</u>: **Big Hearty Salad** (page 237)
- Snack
- <u>Dinner</u>: **Pineapple Chicken Skewers** (page 240) with a side of half a cup of wild rice or quinoa and cooked veggies (e.g., roasted brussels sprouts or sautéed spinach with olive oil and garlic)
- <u>Dessert</u>: Bowl of berries plus two or three squares of dark chocolate

TUESDAY

- <u>Breakfast</u>: **Bowe Glow Berry Smoothie** (page 234)
- <u>Lunch</u>: **Spa Lunch** (page 238)
- Snack
- <u>Dinner</u>: Six or seven ounces of baked wild salmon over two-thirds of a cup of quinoa and unlimited roasted vegetables

- Dessert: One whole fruit (e.g., apple or pear) or a handful of berries plus a small drizzle of honey

WEDNESDAY

- Breakfast: Half a cup of old-fashioned or steel-cut oats cooked with two-thirds of a cup of almond milk and a pinch of cinnamon or pumpkin pie spice, plus a handful of raw walnuts and one tablespoon flaxseeds, sweetened with a drizzle of honey
- Lunch: Open-faced turkey sandwich on a slice of sprouted-grain or multigrain bread with romaine, sliced tomato, and avocado spread or avocado mayo, plus a side salad and a tablespoon of sauerkraut or kimchi
- Snack
- Dinner: Six or seven ounces of pan-seared sole or branzino with a side of roasted brussels sprouts and half a cup of wild rice
- Dessert: **Chocolate Banana Mousse** (page 243)

THURSDAY

- Breakfast: One six-ounce serving of Greek-style yogurt topped with chopped raw nuts and a drizzle of honey plus one slice of multigrain bread topped with mashed avocado and a pinch of salt
- Lunch: Fresh salad greens with raw veggies, topped with grilled or poached salmon and dressed with a handful of pistachios, olive oil, and balsamic vinegar
- Snack
- Dinner: **Hearty Vegetable Dinner Scramble** (page 239) with a side of half a cup of quinoa
- Dessert: **Avocado Mousse** (page 243)

FRIDAY

- Breakfast: **Bowe Glow Berry Smoothie** (page 234)
- Lunch: **Decadent Salad with Spinach, Chicken, Crushed Walnuts, and Sliced Strawberries** (page 238)
- Snack
- Dinner: Six or seven ounces of grilled Chilean sea bass (or, alternatively, grilled chicken breast) topped with one tablespoon miso paste and served with sautéed collard greens and half a cup of quinoa
- Dessert: A cup of fresh berries topped with a scoop of sorbet

SATURDAY

- Breakfast: **Strawberry Banana Overnight Oats** (page 236)
- Lunch: One slice of sprouted-grain bread topped with almond butter and a sliced banana and served with one hard-boiled egg (toast the bread first before adding the banana and nut butter for a warm, gooey treat)
- Snack
- Dinner: **Broiled Honey-Orange-Lemon Chicken** (page 241) over half a cup of whole-grain brown or wild rice, served with sautéed string beans and zucchini (dressed with olive oil or butter made from the milk of grass-fed cows)
- Dessert: One serving of **Rich Avocado Truffles** (page 244)

SUNDAY

- Breakfast: **Bowe Glow Pancakes** (page 237) with **Golden Milk** (page 235)
- Lunch: **Dandelion-Green Smoothie** (page 235)
- Snack

- <u>Dinner</u>: Four or five ounces of grilled steak with **Hearty Roasted Veggie Mix** (page 242)
- <u>Dessert</u>: Two squares of dark chocolate dipped in one tablespoon of almond butter

WEEK 2: FOCUS ON YOUR BRAIN

Now that you've been on the Bowe Glow path for one week, you should be feeling—and looking—a little better. Have your sugar cravings waned? Are you feeling a bit lighter on your feet? Clearer in your skin? Sharper in your mind? More inspired to keep going? In the second week, let's turn to addressing the habits that will support the health (and function) of the brain, which, as you know, is the second link in the gut-brain-skin connection.

I recommend devoting at least one hour per day to stress-reducing strategies. This doesn't mean you always need to carve out one full, uninterrupted hour in the day—you can create your own mix of activities, from yoga, deep-breathing exercises, and even calling a friend to sweating it out in a formal group exercise class. But whether the time is taken all in one shot or broken up throughout the day, schedule it on a calendar and protect it as though it were a business meeting or your child's graduation ceremony. Doctor's orders! If you don't give your body and mind the opportunity to recover, you will break, and so will your skin. Here are some ideas that reinforce the power of exercise, meditation, and sleep—concepts I explored in chapter 7.

Get Moving

Sorry, but you knew this was coming. If you don't already have an exercise routine, it's time to start one. No more couch-potato syndrome. No more excuses to skip exercise. If you've been sedentary, start with five to ten minutes of high-intensity interval exercise (thirty seconds of maximal effort followed by ninety seconds of recovery), eventually working your way up to twenty minutes total (alternating between high and low intensity), at least three times per week. This can be done any number of ways: walking outside and varying your speed and levels of intensity (especially where there are hills), using traditional gym equipment, or following along with an online video and performing a routine in the comfort of your home. Get creative here — and make it fun! That's the most important factor in getting you moving. If the thought of a treadmill has you thinking "dreadmill," guess what: pick something else that motivates you! It's as simple as that.

I can't reiterate this enough: these days, if conventional gyms aren't your thing, opportunities to exercise are everywhere, so there's really no excuse. I don't care which activity you choose. Just pick one! Get out your calendar and schedule your physical activities.

Also plan to move more throughout the day, especially if you have a day during which there's absolutely no time to devote to formal exercise. Think about the ways you can sneak in more minutes of physical activity while at work or home. All the research indicates that the health benefits of three ten-minute bouts of exercise are similar to those of a single thirty-minute workout. So if you are short on time on any given day, just break up your routine into bite-size chunks. And think of ways to combine exercise with other tasks: for example, conduct a meeting with a colleague at work while walking outside, or watch television at night while you complete a set of stretching exercises on the floor. If possible, limit the minutes you spend sitting on your derriere. Walk around, if you can, while you talk on the phone; take the stairs rather than the elevator, and park far away from the front door to your office or home. The more you move throughout the day, the more your body — and skin — benefit.

If you already maintain a fitness regimen, see if you can increase your workouts to a minimum of thirty minutes a day five days a week. This also might be the week you try something different, such as attending a dance class, dropping in on a Pilates studio, or calling a friend who you know is an exercise fiend and asking for help and ideas. It's important that your daily routines are balanced and that you vary your workouts overall so your body's many muscle groups all get attention. The body also responds well to being surprised. When you get used to doing one form of exercise all the time, your body adapts to it. This means its benefits will diminish unless you dial up the intensity each and every time (which most people don't do!). The more you vary your routine, the more you will see and feel your body grow stronger, more toned, and healthier.

So ask yourself: do you monotonously do the same routine every day? Do you have a strong heart because you love your cardio but have no real muscle strength elsewhere? You see, I used to be a "cardio queen." I was convinced that if I wasn't dripping in sweat by the end of my workout, it didn't really count as a workout. I was thin, but I wasn't especially toned, and I didn't feel particularly strong. But more important, I was mentally exhausted and scattered and would find myself craving unhealthful foods just to refuel my energy stores and make it through the day (muffins and baked goods called out to me when I walked into a coffee shop. Okay, they didn't just call out, they jumped up and down, screaming, "Whitney, look at us!"). A knee injury came at just the right time. It forced me to slow down my cardio and try new things, including Pilates. Once I realized how powerful and centered a noncardio workout could make me feel, I began to explore all kinds of exercise.

Here is my current exercise breakdown (note: this may have changed by the time you read this book, because I'm always trying new things!). The take-home message should be obvious: variety and balance.

- Two days per week of strength training (with weights and resistance bands)
- One day per week of cardio intervals (bursts of high-intensity cardio followed by a recovery period, then repeat)
- One day per week of Pilates (fifty minutes)
- One day per week of light cardio (e.g., thirty minutes on the elliptical machine at medium intensity while I watch my favorite show on a tablet)
- One day per week of yoga

Right now, my yoga class is on Friday afternoons, and I look forward to it all week! I end my yoga sessions with a few minutes of Shavasana, a yoga pose that doubles as a form of meditation. I used to come home on Fridays cross-eyed and fatigued. Now I come home refreshed and looking forward to a wonderful weekend with my family. The new variety in my routine keeps my body strong and balanced. My heart is healthy (thanks to my two cardio days), my muscles are strong and powerful (thanks to strength training), and I feel long, lean, and flexible with an incredibly strong core thanks to Pilates and yoga. I'm not saying you have to do what I do. I'm just saying to shoot for balance and variety. Your body and brain will respond better than they would if you did the same type of exercise every day.

Get Quiet

As I explained in chapter 7, meditation is like magic for your body—calming it down quickly and inducing what's called the relaxation response. But you don't have to engage in classic meditation to achieve the same effects. You can practice deep breathing, tai chi, or kundalini yoga, which is a style of yoga with meditative aspects. Your goal is to find a time during every day to press Pause and trigger that relaxation response. At the very least, try to establish a daily practice at the same time every day this week. Maybe it's first thing in the morning, after lunch, at precisely 3:00 p.m. (set your alarm on your smartphone), or before bed. I don't care when. I care that you do it!

Get Your Beauty Sleep

In addition to establishing meditation strategies and better exercise habits, use week 2 to focus on your sleep hygiene. If you get less than six hours of sleep per night, you can start by increasing that period of time to at least seven hours. For most people, this is the bare minimum if you want to have normal, healthful levels of fluctuating hormones in your body that are matched to a healthful circadian rhythm. Some people can get by on less sleep, but the vast majority of us would do well to bank seven hours a night. And remember that if you don't get enough sleep at night, it undoes the benefits you gained from the exercise you did that day. Here are my top three tips for getting a good night's sleep, a refresher course on the material I presented in chapter 7.

Protect your sleep time as if it were a prized possession. Go to bed and get up at roughly the same time daily no matter what. Keep your bedtime routine consistent; it might include downtime, tooth-brushing, a warm bath — whatever you need to do to wind down and signal your body that it's time for sleep. Also, don't forget to keep your bedroom quiet, cool, dark, and electronics-free.

Plan your last meal of the day. Leave at least two hours between dinnertime and bedtime so your stomach is settled and poised for you to go to sleep. If you need a bedtime snack, save your dessert for thirty minutes to an hour before bedtime.

Mind those uppers and downers. Caffeine and alcohol will work against you at bedtime. Make sure that if you consume these ingredients, you do so smartly and not within three hours of bedtime. Stop drinking caffeinated beverages (including tea) by midafternoon. Alcohol may make you feel sleepy initially, but as it metabolizes in the body it can trigger wakefulness. Don't have a second glass of wine, or maybe even skip alcohol in the evening altogether—at least during these three weeks.

By the time you reach the end of the second week, you should be feeling even better than you did after the first. But don't panic if you don't feel like you've totally hit your stride yet. Most of us have at least one weak spot in our lives that requires extra attention. Perhaps finding the time to exercise is exceedingly challenging given the demands placed on you, or you're the type who has a hard time evicting carbs that you know your body—and skin—don't love. Use this upcoming third week to find a rhythm in your new routine. Solidify your new habits and beauty patterns. It is said to take only three weeks to get into the groove of establishing new habits. That's not a long time, given the payoffs. Identify areas in your life where you struggle to maintain this protocol and see what you can do to rectify that in week 3.

WEEK 3: FOCUS ON YOUR SKIN

Now that your skin is on the road to radiant from the inside out, this week it's time to work from the outside in. Refer back to chapter 8 for the details of proper skin care. Below are instructional outlines of the new routines I hope you establish this week, starting with a list of to-dos.

Skin-Prep Checklist
- Clean up your bathroom by removing harsh cleansers, and soaps, loofahs, body scrubbers, sponges, and old cosmetics. Replace them

with new products that meet my guidelines (see chapter 8 and go to my website for brand recommendations)

- Toss any soaps that say "antibacterial" on the packaging
- Limit use of hand sanitizers—*only* use them when gentle soap and water are not available
- Toss any alcohol-based toners or astringents
- If you've been taking a topical antibiotic (such as erythromycin or clindamycin) for a skin condition, make sure you are also using a topical benzoyl peroxide to limit bacterial resistance issues. Better yet, ask your dermatologist for antibiotic-free topical prescriptions or OTC alternatives. With any luck, if you follow all the guidelines in this book, you will soon find yourself no longer needing prescriptions. But sometimes you need a dermatologist's help to get you to that point.
- If you've been taking an oral antibiotic for a chronic skin condition, make sure you are also taking an oral probiotic (you should have started this during the first week, so this is just a reminder). Also, make sure you don't use oral antibiotics for longer than three months! If your condition is not significantly improved after three months of taking an oral antibiotic, work with your dermatologist on an alternative strategy.
- Purchase at least one probiotic-infused topical product and start using it this week as directed on the packaging. Go to my website for brand suggestions tailored to your skin issue. I also recommend that you choose one day this week to apply a probiotic-rich mask on your face. Choose another day to try a mask rich in coconut oil. See my recipes on page 244.
- Purchase your skin-care products:
  - Moisturizing body wash or bar
  - Facial cleanser
  - Daytime serum rich in antioxidants—choose one that's formulated for the face, neck, and chest, and try to find one con-

taining vitamins C, E, ferulic acid, pomegranate, zinc, copper, or green tea. It's unlikely you'll find any single product that has all these ingredients (if you do, please let me know), so go with the one that has most of them and is packaged well (no clear bottles, because exposure to light can degrade these sensitive ingredients)

○ Moisturizer with sunscreen

○ Nighttime serum—look for one that contains ingredients targeted to your concerns. For example, there are serums that target fine lines and wrinkles, serums that address dark spots, and even serums that can prevent acne flares. If you don't have any specific issues to address and are looking for just a general night serum, I recommend one that contains peptides, growth factors, antioxidants, and retinol (again, see my website for brand ideas). You can also buy a stand-alone retinol product and use it sporadically rather than every night to avoid unpleasant side effects—see chapter 8 for details; not everyone can tolerate daily use of a retinol product

○ Nighttime moisturizing cream

The Bowe Glow Morning Routine

When cleansing your body in the shower or bath, you don't need fancy brushes or loofahs. In fact you would do well to use your bare hands and a moisturizing body wash or bar. Look for a wash or bar that is soap- and fragrance-free if you suffer from eczema or allergies. Ideally, use one that incorporates moisturizers or claims to leave the skin hydrated (look for the words *hydrating* or *moisturizing* on the label). Bathe with warm water, not water so hot that it leaves you itchy and dried out.

You can cleanse your face either in the shower or bath or afterward.

For your morning routine, find a gentle, pH-balanced, soap-free hydrating skin cleanser that is water-based. Look for words like *gentle, nonirritating,* and *mild.* A cleanser that can be used on babies or is designed for special-needs skin is usually a solid product.

When washing your face, use lukewarm water and your fingertips only. Pat dry. Up to twice weekly, you can exfoliate your face with a cleanser and a gentle scrub or with a chemical scrub that contains ingredients such as glycolic acid and lactic acid (see page 168 for rules of exfoliation). Doing this more than twice a week can compromise the skin's barrier, resulting in redness, blotchiness, sensitivity to other skin-care products, and accelerated aging.

Before you apply anything else to your face, apply an antioxidant serum. (Alternatively, you can add a few drops of an antioxidant serum to your sunscreen.)

Next, apply your daily sunscreen-containing moisturizer — or your moisturizing sunscreen. Yes, your sunscreen can double as a moisturizer; if you add a few drops of an antioxidant serum to your sunscreen, you've got a triple threat.

Finally, apply your makeup, if you choose to wear it. Many women are afraid of makeup when they shouldn't be. Makeup does more good than harm (it's confidence- and beauty-boosting!). You don't want to use anything too heavy, such as an oil-based foundation. Look for the word *noncomedogenic,* meaning it won't clog pores. Use quality, nationally recognized brands that have done their testing. These are the brands that take up a lot of real estate in large drugstore chains and department stores. Although drugstore cosmetics are often just as good as those sold at department stores, sometimes it's fun to splurge a little bit and go for more expensive products. I, for example, like a brand of foundation found only in department and specialty makeup stores because I like how it feels on my skin.

Also note: there's a lot of unnecessary fear surrounding chemicals in products and whether or not organic is the way to go. At the same time, we read frightening headlines about beauty-care products whose chemicals and detergents end up causing serious side effects, from rashes to hair loss, even though they're often sold as better alternatives to traditional products. Just because something is organic doesn't necessarily mean that it's safe or that it won't trigger a reaction. Remember: anthrax and poison ivy are natural and organic! Whether you're buying organic cosmetics or not, go with brands that have a solid reputation and are not plagued by bad press. You can use the "Dr. Whitney's Picks" section of my website as your launching pad.

The Bowe Glow Evening Routine

Nighttime is when your skin should refresh and renew itself, recovering from the free radicals, pollution, and stressors it encounters during the day. You want to give your skin everything it needs for powerful healing at night.

If you've been wearing eye makeup or heavy or long-wear foundation, or if you live in or near a city (where pollution rates are high), I recommend double cleansing. This means using an oil-based cleanser followed by a gentle water-based cleanser. There are great oil-based cleansers on the market, or you can make your own using olive oil (see below). If you're not a big makeup person and don't live in a city, you can just use the same water-based cleanser you used in the morning.

DIY Makeup Remover

In a bottle with an airtight top, place two cups of filtered water. Then add two tablespoons of olive oil. Shake the mixture well before using. Apply to your face with cotton pads.

Within five minutes of washing your face, be sure to trap the moisture onto your skin by applying some nighttime products. Start with your retinol product if you're using one. If your serum contains retinol, you don't need a separate retinol product; avoid doubling up on the retinol application.

Dab a pea-size amount on your forehead, cheeks, nose, and chin, then rub it in. That one pea-size squirt should cover your entire face. Then dab a second pea-size amount across your neck and chest. You may not feel like you're getting enough, but tiny little microscopic bits of ingredients will migrate all over your face, neck, and chest. Plus, at the beginning, you really want to err on the side of "less is more."

Next apply your serum and night cream on top of the retinoid product to seal it in and prevent dryness and irritation. Use a night cream that has hydrating ingredients such as hyaluronic acid, vitamins, and peptides.

Ease a Visible Skin Condition with Evening Primrose Oil

Anyone who has a visible skin condition such as acne, psoriasis, rosacea, or eczema should try a topical application of evening primrose oil. This is a great source of linoleic acid, a beneficial fatty acid that can reduce inflammation in the skin. Apply this between your serum and night cream.

If you live in a place where harsh winters dry out your skin, use an eye cream or coconut oil around your eyes during those months (some people like to use eye creams throughout the year, no matter where they live — that's fine, too). You can also apply coconut oil to your legs from the knee down as well as to your heels, since there aren't a lot of oil glands there. The elbow and knee scrub on page 171 works well for these areas. On nights when you have extra time, try a facial mask tailored to your skin's needs (see below for my antioxidant power mask; see page 244 for more).

My Cranberry-Apple Antioxidant Face Mask

One of my favorite power-packed antioxidant skin masks is simple and easy to make but will leave your face feeling radiant and renewed! Cranberries and apples are rich in wrinkle-fighting antioxidants, including vitamin C, which helps collagen production and strengthens your hair and nails. Almond oil is packed with vitamin E, which softens and smooths the skin, improves tone and complexion, and has been shown to slow down the visible signs of aging.

1 apple, peeled, cored, and chopped
½ cup fresh or defrosted frozen cranberries
1 tablespoon almond oil

Combine all ingredients in a food processor until the mixture reaches a pastelike consistency. It should be a bit thick. Spread on clean skin. Leave on for 3–5 minutes, then rinse off with warm water.

If you suffer from a skin disorder that has not been remedied (or not remedied to your liking) by the end of this week, schedule a visit to the dermatologist. How do you find one? Start by asking your friends and coworkers for recommendations. Or ask your internist for a referral.

UH-OH — NOW WHAT?

What do you do after the three weeks are up? You keep doing what you're doing. Aim to stick to my dietary protocol, keep those good lifestyle habits of movement, meditation, and sound sleep, and treat your skin gently every day. Each weekend, plan the week ahead. Set aside ten minutes (or less!) to plan upcoming meals, organize your grocery list, and determine whether you need other supplies, such as a replacement for a night cream that is getting low. See if you can predict the days when you'll be extra harried and prepare for them as best you can. When eating in restaurants, try to choose those that use fresh, organic, and locally grown ingredients. Just as you would prepare your meals at home with whole, fresh, unprocessed ingredients, you'll want to patronize restaurants that do the same. If you buy prepared foods at markets, a practice you should keep to a minimum, look for fresh ingredients free of artificial sweeteners and hydrogenated fats. Keep in mind that if you didn't make it, you simply do not know what is in it.

There are lots of apps now that can help you with your goals, including those that track your movements, help you make smart decisions at the market (e.g., tell you the GI index of various foods), help you meditate by means of guided imagery, and even show you how well you are sleeping at night. Don't be afraid to use technology when it can serve a real purpose and benefit you. I use Google Calendar to help me keep track of my commitments and carve out time to exercise, MyFitnessPal to track my daily diet and favorite recipes, and Breethe to guide me in meditation. Use what works for you.

As I tell my patients, be flexible but consistent. We all have bad days, nights when we don't sleep well, and moments of weakness when we reach for that pastry or second helping of a decadent dessert. Just don't beat yourself up. A slip here or there will not ruin you and your skin. You can recover. If you're consistent for 90 percent of the time, you will be fine. In fact you'll be *better* than fine. Those little slips make us human and help us feel alive.

As doctors learn more about dermatological science, I'll keep you up to date. Just keep checking my website for all the latest and greatest. Nobody expects you to research or test every product out there. That's what I'm here for! Keep the big picture in sight, and remember: the Bowe Glow is within reach. Always. And I'll be right there with you as you proceed. Now, get glowing!

CHAPTER 11

Recipes

Meals and Masks to Get Your Bowe Glow On

THE BOWE GLOW MEALS

Below you'll find recipes for foods and beverages that are suggested in the sample menu on page 217. You do not have to follow that menu plan exactly. Feel free to create your own dishes using the guidelines outlined in the book. The goal is to focus on whole, fresh, unprocessed foods that are as close to nature as possible. Remember, when buying food, go organic, grass-fed, and/or wild whenever possible.

BEVERAGES

Bowe Glow Berry Smoothie   SERVES 1

⅔ cup unsweetened almond milk

1 tablespoon marine collagen protein powder or a plant-based protein powder

½ avocado, peeled and pitted

2–3 dried dates, pitted

½ cup frozen berries

1 teaspoon vanilla extract

1 teaspoon cinnamon

Handful of ice cubes

Place all ingredients in a blender and blend until smooth (about 45 seconds). Add more ice cubes if the smoothie is not cold or thick enough.

Dandelion-Green Smoothie · SERVES 1

1 cup filtered water

1 cup chopped dandelion greens

1 banana

1 cup fresh or frozen berries

1 tablespoon marine collagen protein powder or a plant-based protein powder

1 tablespoon honey or a pinch of powdered stevia

Pinch of cinnamon

Place all ingredients except cinnamon in a blender and blend until smooth (about 45 seconds). Pour into a tall glass and top with cinnamon.

Golden Milk   SERVES 1

⅔ cup unsweetened almond milk

1 (3-inch) cinnamon stick

1 tablespoon honey

1 tablespoon coconut oil

¼ teaspoon whole black peppercorns

½ teaspoon powdered turmeric

1 (1-inch) piece fresh ginger, peeled and thinly sliced

1 cup filtered water

Pinch of cinnamon

Combine all ingredients except cinnamon in a medium saucepan and place over medium-high heat. Whisk until smooth. Then bring the mixture to a low boil. Reduce heat and simmer until flavors are blended, about 15 minutes. Strain the mixture into a mug and top with a pinch of cinnamon. You can keep golden milk in the fridge for about 4 days.

Detox Water   MAKES ABOUT 8 SERVINGS

1 pitcher filtered water (at least 60 ounces)

Juice of 1 lemon

1 lemon, thinly sliced

¼ cup fresh mint leaves

20 fresh blackberries, smashed into a pulp

1 cucumber, thinly sliced

Combine all the ingredients and chill in the refrigerator.

BREAKFASTS

Strawberry Banana Overnight Oats   SERVES 2

1 cup rolled oats

1 tablespoon chia seeds

2 teaspoons pure maple syrup

¾ cup unsweetened almond milk (see note)

¼ cup unsweetened coconut milk (see note)

1 scoop plant-based protein powder (vanilla or unflavored)

½ cup fresh sliced strawberries

½ banana, sliced on the diagonal

Handful of slivered almonds

Pinch of cinnamon

Mix the oats, chia seeds, maple syrup, almond milk, coconut milk, and protein powder in a small bowl. Divide mixture into two mason jars. Cover and allow to sit overnight in the refrigerator. In the morning, stir each jar to make the mixture nice and creamy. Top with strawberries, banana, slivered almonds, and cinnamon.

Note: *You can substitute an almond milk–coconut milk blend for the two separate milks if desired.*

Bowe Glow Pancakes   SERVES 2

1 cup almond flour

1 teaspoon baking soda

Pinch salt

½ ripe banana, mashed

2 eggs

¼ cup almond milk

2 teaspoons vanilla extract

1–2 tablespoons ghee

2 tablespoons almond butter (optional)

In a medium mixing bowl, whisk the almond flour, baking soda, and salt. In a separate bowl, whisk the mashed banana, eggs, almond milk, and vanilla extract. Pour the dry ingredients into the wet and mix until smooth. Preheat a griddle or frying pan on medium-low heat and add the ghee. Drop 2 table-spoons batter into the pan to form pancakes and cook 3–4 minutes on each side, or until golden. Transfer pancakes to warmed serving plates and keep warm in a low oven while you cook the rest of the batter. Top with almond butter if desired and serve with Golden Milk (page 235).

SALADS AND LUNCHES

Big Hearty Salad   SERVES 1

For the salad

2 cups mixed baby greens

1 vine-ripe tomato, chopped

½ cucumber, peeled and sliced

1 red or green bell pepper, seeded, deveined, and sliced

1 cup broccoli florets

2 fresh figs, chopped

3 ounces sliced organic roasted chicken or wild-caught cooked fish

Handful of raw nuts or seeds

For the balsamic vinaigrette (makes about 1 cup)

¼ cup balsamic vinegar

2 cloves garlic, chopped

½ shallot, chopped

1 tablespoon Dijon mustard

1 tablespoon fresh rosemary leaves

Juice of 1 lemon

1 teaspoon salt

½ teaspoon ground black pepper

½ cup extra-virgin olive oil

Combine salad ingredients in a large bowl. To make the dressing, whisk together the vinegar, garlic, shallot, mustard, rosemary, lemon juice, salt, and pepper in a medium bowl, then slowly drizzle in the olive oil, whisking constantly. Add 2–3 tablespoons of dressing to the salad and toss. Store leftover vinaigrette in a tightly covered container in the refrigerator.

Decadent Salad with Spinach, Chicken, Crushed Walnuts, and Sliced Strawberries   SERVES 1

1–2 cups fresh baby spinach

⅔ cup raw dandelion greens, chopped

3 ounces boneless skinless grilled chicken, diced

1 tablespoon crumbled feta cheese

1 cup sliced strawberries

¼ cup crushed raw walnuts

2 tablespoons balsamic vinaigrette (see above)

Toss all ingredients in a mixing bowl and transfer to a plate.

Spa Lunch   SERVES 1

1 cup chopped raw vegetables, such as cauliflower, onion, mushrooms, and bell pepper

3 tablespoons extra-virgin olive oil, divided

1 teaspoon powdered turmeric

1 tablespoon chopped fresh oregano or 1 teaspoon dried oregano

Pinch of salt

1 cup uncooked quinoa, rinsed

6 ounces wild salmon

1 tablespoon spicy brown mustard (optional)

To make the roasted vegetables

Preheat the oven to 350°F. Combine the chopped vegetables in a large bowl. Add 2 tablespoons extra-virgin olive oil plus the turmeric, oregano, and salt. Mix with your hands, then arrange the veggies in a roasting pan and roast for 45 minutes, tossing midway through cooking time. Leave the oven on for the salmon.

To make the quinoa

Combine the quinoa and 2 cups water in a medium saucepan. Bring to a boil. Reduce the heat to low, cover, and simmer until tender and most of the liquid has been absorbed, 15–20 minutes. Fluff with a fork.

To make the salmon

Place the fish on a baking sheet lined with foil. Coat the salmon lightly with the remaining olive oil and bake for 10 minutes. If desired, top with a thin layer of spicy brown mustard and broil for 1 minute, or until browned.

Place the cooked fish on top of the quinoa, surround with the cooked veggies, and serve.

DINNERS

Hearty Vegetable Dinner Scramble   SERVES 1

1 small onion, diced

1 bell pepper, seeded, deveined, and diced

1 cup chopped fresh baby spinach

¼ cup sliced mushrooms

4 egg whites

1 whole egg

Salt and ground black pepper to taste

1 teaspoon pesto or salsa (optional)

Coat a medium frying pan with extra-virgin-olive-oil cooking spray. Sauté the onion until softened, about 2 minutes. Add the remaining vegetables and sauté until crisp-tender, about 5 minutes. Beat the egg whites and egg in a small bowl, then add to the vegetables. Scramble together until the eggs are fully cooked. Season and top with pesto or salsa, if desired.

Pineapple Chicken Skewers   SERVES 2

For the marinade
¼ cup freshly squeezed lemon juice

½ teaspoon salt

½ teaspoon ground black pepper

½ teaspoon hot red pepper flakes

4 strips lemon peel

3 cloves garlic, minced

½ cup chopped fresh parsley

2 tablespoons chopped fresh basil

2 tablespoons chopped fresh dill

½ cup extra-virgin olive oil

For the chicken
2 boneless skinless chicken breasts, cut into 1-inch cubes

½ fresh pineapple, peeled, cored, and cut into 1-inch chunks

1 large red bell pepper, seeded, deveined, and cut into 1-inch chunks

1 large yellow bell pepper, seeded, deveined, and cut into 1-inch chunks

1 large red onion, cut into 1-inch chunks

4 bamboo skewers

In a medium mixing bowl, combine the lemon juice, salt, black pepper, and red pepper flakes and whisk until the salt crystals are dissolved. Add the lemon peel, garlic, parsley, basil, and dill. Gradually whisk in the olive oil.

Place the chicken in a resealable plastic bag and add the marinade. Seal the bag and gently shake to mix. Refrigerate for at least an hour or overnight.

Soak the bamboo skewers in water for 25 minutes.

Preheat the grill to medium.

Thread alternating pieces of chicken, pineapple, bell pepper, and onion onto each skewer. Grill 4–5 minutes on each side, or until the chicken is fully cooked and the vegetables are crisp-tender. Alternatively, preheat the broiler. Arrange the threaded skewers on a broiler pan and broil 4 inches from heat source for 4–5 minutes on each side. Serve immediately.

Broiled Honey-Orange-Lemon Chicken SERVES 4

2 tablespoons extra-virgin olive oil

¼ cup honey

¼ cup freshly squeezed lemon juice

Several pinches of sea salt or pink Himalayan salt

1 teaspoon finely grated lemon zest

Pinch of ground black pepper

4 boneless skinless chicken breasts

4 orange slices

In a large mixing bowl, combine all ingredients except the chicken and orange slices. Place the chicken in a shallow baking dish and pour the marinade over it. Cover and refrigerate at least 2 hours or overnight.

Preheat the broiler. Remove the chicken breasts from the baking dish, reserving marinade, and place breasts on a broiler pan. Arrange the orange slices over the top. Broil 4 inches from heat source for 10 minutes, then brush with the reserved marinade, turn the breasts over, and broil 10 more minutes. Continue to broil until chicken starts to brown, 5–10 additional minutes, or until you pierce it with a fork and the juices run clear. Strain the hot marinade over the chicken and serve.

SNACKS

Savory Avo-Yogurt Dip   SERVES 2

1 ripe avocado, peeled and pitted

½ cup plain Greek-style yogurt

¼ cup cilantro leaves

1 tablespoon chopped white onion

1 tablespoon freshly squeezed lime juice

Pinch of salt

¼ teaspoon ground black pepper

Puree all ingredients in a food processor. Serve with fresh veggies as an appetizer or snack.

Hearty Roasted Veggie Mix 1   SERVES 2

1 whole garlic bulb, unpeeled

2 tablespoons extra-virgin olive oil

4 small yellow onions, halved

6 fresh plum tomatoes, halved

3 zucchini, sliced into spears

Salt and ground black pepper to taste

Preheat oven to 350°F. Slice ½ inch off the top of the garlic bulb and wrap the bulb in foil. Combine remaining ingredients in a large bowl and toss. Arrange the veggies in a roasting pan and add the garlic bulb. Roast for 25 minutes, or until the veggies are tender. Squeeze garlic pulp from the baked cloves over the vegetables and mix well. Adjust seasonings if desired.

Hearty Roasted Veggie Mix 2   SERVES 2

1 whole garlic bulb, separated into cloves and peeled

2 tablespoons extra-virgin olive oil

⅔ cup broccoli florets

⅔ cup cauliflower florets

⅔ cup sliced mushrooms

4–5 asparagus spears, cut into 1-inch pieces

1 small onion, cut into 1-inch chunks

2 tablespoons fresh rosemary leaves

Salt and ground black pepper to taste

Preheat oven to 350°F. Combine ingredients in a large bowl and toss. Arrange the veggies in a roasting pan and roast for 45 minutes, or until the veggies are tender and golden brown. Adjust seasonings if desired.

DESSERTS

Avocado Mousse   SERVES 1–2

1 large ripe avocado, peeled and pitted

¼ cup unsweetened cocoa powder

¼ cup unsweetened almond or coconut milk

2 teaspoons stevia

1 teaspoon vanilla extract

Handful of berries or 1 ounce cacao nibs

Puree the avocado in a food processor until smooth. Mix the cocoa powder and milk until combined, then add to the avocado. Stir in the stevia and vanilla extract and transfer the mousse to individual serving bowls. Chill for 30 minutes. When ready to eat, top with berries or cacao nibs.

Chocolate Banana Mousse   SERVES 1

1 peeled banana, frozen

2 tablespoons unsweetened cocoa powder

Splash of unsweetened almond or coconut milk

1 tablespoon marine collagen protein powder or plant-based protein powder

1 tablespoon honey or pinch of stevia (optional)

Combine all ingredients in a blender and blend until smooth.

Rich Avocado Truffles   MAKES 10 TRUFFLES

4 ounces dark chocolate, at least 70% cacao, coarsely chopped

1–2 ripe avocados, peeled, pitted, and mashed

Pinch of salt

2 tablespoons unsweetened cocoa powder

Melt the chocolate in a heatproof bowl over a pot of boiling water. Remove bowl from heat and mix in the avocado and salt. Combine well—the mixture should be quite thick. Cover the bowl and chill until the mixture can be rolled into balls, about 1 hour. Sprinkle the cocoa powder on a piece of wax paper. Use a melon baller or a spoon to form the truffles into ¾-inch balls. Roll each truffle in cocoa powder, then arrange them in a single layer on a serving plate or dish. Refrigerate until ready to serve.

THE BOWE GLOW MASKS

Try one of these probiotic-rich and coconut-oil masks at least once a week. As I suggest in chapter 10, go for a probiotic mask one night a week and choose a mask containing coconut oil on another night. Even though I've noted which masks are ideal for certain skin conditions, there's nothing wrong with trying all of them to see which one or two you enjoy the most and which produces the best results. Sometimes a little experimentation is just what the doctor ordered. Find the go-to mask that leaves your skin glowing, hydrated, and feeling great.

Probiotic Power Mask with Turmeric and Honey for Dull Skin Prone to the Big Four

Note that turmeric can leave a slight stain on the skin if not combined in the right ratio with other ingredients or if left on the skin too long.

1 teaspoon organic turmeric powder

1 teaspoon raw organic honey

1 tablespoon organic plain (unflavored) kefir

In a small bowl, combine all ingredients. Apply to clean skin and let sit for 8–10 minutes. Rinse with warm water and a soft washcloth. Pat dry. Moisturize as usual.

Probiotic Power Mask with Jojoba Oil and Honey for Acne, Psoriasis, and Sunburn

1 teaspoon jojoba oil

1 teaspoon raw organic honey

2–3 capsules probiotics (see page 104 for recommendations)

In a small bowl, combine the jojoba oil and raw honey. Open the probiotics capsules, empty the contents into the bowl, and mix well. Apply to clean skin and let sit for 15–20 minutes, then rinse with warm water and a soft washcloth. Pat dry. Moisturize with a skin-balancing oil, such as rose-hip-seed oil, immediately afterward.

Probiotic Power Mask for Depuffing and Exfoliating

The caffeine in coffee grounds helps to reduce swelling and puffiness. The yogurt, in addition to containing probiotics, acts as a soothing emollient. The coconut oil adds moisture. If you don't add the coconut oil, make sure to follow the mask with a moisturizer.

3 tablespoons plain Greek-style yogurt

2 tablespoons finely ground coffee

1 tablespoon coconut oil (optional)

In a bowl, combine the yogurt, coffee, and coconut oil, if desired, mixing together with a fork until you have a paste. Apply to clean skin using a gentle circular motion. Let sit for 20 minutes, then rinse with warm water and a soft washcloth. Pat dry.

Green Tea and Honey Power Mask for Combating Redness

The green tea in this mask is soothing, removes impurities, and reduces inflammation. The honey is antibacterial and soothing, and the coconut oil adds moisture.

> 2 bags green tea
> Warm water
> 3 tablespoons honey
> 1 tablespoon coconut oil (optional)

Cut open the tea bags and empty their contents into a small bowl. Add a few drops of water and mix with a fork just to dampen. Then add the honey and coconut oil, if desired, and mix with the fork. Apply the mask to clean skin. Let sit for 15–20 minutes, then rinse with warm water and a soft washcloth. Pat dry.

Oatmeal Coconut-Oil Power Mask for Sensitive Skin

This mask is great for people who cannot tolerate scrubs or other exfoliating formulas, including people who have eczema, acne, or rosacea. The oatmeal gently removes the dead cells on the surface to reveal glowing skin underneath; melting the coconut oil results in the best consistency.

> 1 tablespoon coconut oil
> 3 tablespoons rolled oats
> Warm water

Melt the coconut oil in a microwave or on the stove and set aside. Place the oatmeal in a small bowl and slowly pour in enough warm water to create a pastelike consistency. Add the coconut oil and mix well. Apply the mask to clean skin and exfoliate by gently rubbing in a circular motion. Leave the mask on for 15 minutes. Rinse with cool water and pat dry. Moisturize as usual.

Coconut-Oil Mask with Avocado for Dry Skin

¼ ripe avocado, peeled and pitted

½ teaspoon powdered nutmeg

1 tablespoon coconut oil

In a small bowl, mash the avocado with a fork. Mix in the nutmeg and coconut oil to form a paste. Apply to clean skin and leave on for 10–15 minutes. Rinse with cold water and pat dry. Moisturize as usual.

Acknowledgments

I have been inspired, encouraged, and mentored by so many incredible minds along my journey. I cannot possibly list all the people — teachers, students, friends, peers, and mentors — who have touched my life and who have made this dream a reality. Although I will keep my remarks short and sweet, I will be forever grateful to each of you.

First I want to thank my patients for teaching me more than any textbook ever did. You each touch my heart every day and inspire me to continue to learn and evolve.

I also want to thank my research mentors, Dr. David Margolis and the late Dr. Alan Shalita, who encouraged me to trust my instincts and explore alternative theories, including natural, sustainable treatments for skin disease. This book is the culmination of the work we started more than a decade ago, and I am so proud to share it with you.

Thanks also to the impeccably talented team at Little, Brown: I feel so blessed to have worked with the brightest, most capable minds in the world of publishing. Kristin Loberg, you are an absolute artist with words, and I am forever grateful for the many hours you spent assisting me in translating the most complicated scientific concepts into empowering text that will bring the gift of health through knowledge to so many. I can't imagine doing any of this without Bonnie Solow, my literary agent, by my side. You have exceeded my expectations every step of the way, from helping cultivate the initial concept to guiding our team throughout the entire publication process with your clear vision and deepest wisdom. Tracy Behar, you just *got* the book from day one. Your experience, coupled with your intuition, made the entire process a joy for everyone on your team. And thank you to the entire Little, Brown crew: Zea Moscone, Pamela Brown, Lauren Velasquez, Betsy Uhrig, Ian Straus, and Elora Weil. It has been both a pleasure and an honor to work with such a talented group of people.

Of course I also want to express my gratitude to my family: Josh, thank you for your unwavering and passionate support and for filling our home with laughter and love; Doran, my beloved sister and partner, I would not be who I am without your guidance, love, and support; Mom, thank you for making me believe the sky is the limit.

Doran, your tireless work in every facet of our partnership deserves a few more words at minimum. I don't believe it's possible to love and trust another individual as completely as I do you. Your opinion is invaluable to my every decision, and you make me laugh and enjoy every minute of our journey. I feel so blessed to have a partner and sister who shares my dreams both professionally and personally and who has always embraced my ideas and my passion with open arms and an open mind. Your dance moves are simply the icing on the cake of our bond, which enriches my mind, my heart, and my soul.

To Dr. Joshua Fox and my Advanced Dermatology family: thank you for creating a home for me at our practice and for supporting me while I open the doors of that home to our patients. I feel incredibly valued, and as a result I am able to deliver the best to my patients and offer them everything I possibly can as a physician and advocate.

I also cannot imagine having undertaken this journey without my father, the resilient and compassionate Dr. Frank Bowe, whom we lost too young. As a passionate disability rights advocate, thought leader, and innovator, he taught me to look past perceived limitations, to push boundaries, and to truly see the person behind a disability, disorder, or ailment. His mind-set and philosophy continue to guide and inspire me long after his passing, and I could not be more proud to follow in his footsteps as a published author.

Finally I would like to thank you, my readers, who have made a decision to enrich yourselves with the information in this book, which I know will change not only your skin but also your overall health, your outlook, your energy levels, and, quite possibly, key aspects of your daily life. I have enjoyed our journey through these pages together!

Notes

The following is a list of books, scientific papers, and Web citations that might be helpful if you want to learn more about some of the ideas and concepts presented in the preceding chapters. For updated information and access to new insights, please visit www.DrWhitneyBowe .com.

Introduction: Learning to Love Your Good Bugs

1. W. P. Bowe, S. S. Joshi, and A. R. Shalita, "Diet and Acne," *Journal of the American Academy of Dermatology* 63, no. 1 (July 2010): 124–41.
2. J. L. St. Sauver, et al., "Why Patients Visit Their Doctors: Assessing the Most Prevalent Conditions in a Defined American Population," *Mayo Clinic Proceedings* 88, no. 1 (January 2013): 56–67.
3. See the statistics on the American Academy of Dermatology website at https://www.aad.org/media/stats/conditions.
4. J. G. Muzic, et al., "Incidence and Trends of Basal Cell Carcinoma and Cutaneous Squamous Cell Carcinoma: A Population-Based Study in Olmsted County, Minnesota, 2000 to 2010," *Mayo Clinic Proceedings* 92, no. 6 (June 2017): 890–98.
5. The exact percentage of antibiotics prescriptions written by dermatologists is difficult to assess. This figure is based on unpublished pharmaceuticals industry monitoring data. For more, see John Jesitus's article "Dermatologists Contribute to Overuse of Antibiotics" for the *Dermatology Times* (October 1, 2013) at http://dermatologytimes.modern medicine.com/dermatology-times/content/tags/acne/dermatologists -contribute-overuse-antibiotics.

Chapter 1: Nature's Hidden Secret to Great Skin

1. For updated statistics and facts about skin conditions, go to the American Academy of Dermatology's "Stats and Facts" resource page at https://www.aad.org/media/stats.

2. C. Pontes Tde, et al., "Incidence of Acne Vulgaris in Young Adult Users of Protein-Calorie Supplements in the City of João Pessoa, PB," *Anais brasileiros de ginecologia* 88, no. 6 (November–December 2013): 907–12; C. L. LaRosa, et al., "Consumption of Dairy in Teenagers with and without Acne," *Journal of the American Academy of Dermatology* 75, no. 2 (August 2016): 318–22.

3. M. G. Dominguez-Bello, et al., "Partial Restoration of the Microbiota of Cesarean-Born Infants via Vaginal Microbial Transfer," *Nature Medicine* 22, no. 3 (March 2016): 250–53; M. J. Blaser and M. G. Dominguez-Bello, "The Human Microbiome before Birth," *Cell Host Microbe* 20, no. 5 (2016): 558–60.

4. T. C. Bosch and M. J. McFall-Ngai, "Metaorganisms as the New Frontier," *Zoology* (Jena) 114, no. 4 (September 2011): 185–90.

5. H. E. Blum, "The Human Microbiome," *Advances in Medical Science* 62, no. 2 (July 2017): 414–20; A. B. Shreiner, J. Y. Kao, and V. B. Young, "The Gut Microbiome in Health and in Disease," *Current Opinion in Gastroenterology* 31, no. 1 (January 2015): 69–75.

6. M. Levy, et al., "Dysbiosis and the Immune System," *Nature Reviews: Immunology* 17, no. 4 (April 2017): 219–32; M. M. Kober and W. P. Bowe, "The Effect of Probiotics on Immune Regulation, Acne, and Photoaging," *International Journal of Women's Dermatology* 2, no. 1 (April 2015): 85–89.

7. A. K. DeGruttola, et al., "Current Understanding of Dysbiosis in Disease in Human and Animal Models," *Inflammatory Bowel Diseases* 22, no. 5 (May 2016): 1137–50.

8. J. I. Gordon, et al., "Gut Microbiota from Twins Discordant for Obesity Modulate Metabolism in Mice," *Science* 341, no. 6150 (September 2013): 1079; J. I. Gordon, "Honor Thy Gut Symbionts Redux," *Science* 336, no. 6086 (2012): 1251–1253; J. Xu and J. I. Gordon, "Honor Thy Symbionts," *Proceedings of the National Academy of Sciences of the United States of America* 100, no. 18 (2003): 10452–10459; P. J. Turnbaugh, et al., "The Human Microbiome Project," *Nature* 449, no. 7164 (2007): 804–10; P. J. Turnbaugh, et al., "An Obesity-Associated Gut Microbiome with Increased Capacity for Energy Harvest," *Nature* 444, no. 7122 (2006): 1027–31.

9. P. C. Arck et al., "Neuroimmunology of Stress: Skin Takes Center Stage," *Journal of Investigative Dermatology* 126, no. 8 (August 2006): 1697–1704; A. T. Slominski, et al., "Key Role of CRF in the Skin Stress Response System," *Endocrine Reviews* 34, no. 6 (December 2013): 827–84.

10. C. L. Ventola, "The Antibiotic Resistance Crisis: Part 1: Causes and Threats," *Pharmacy & Therapeutics* 40, no. 4 (April 2015): 277–83; C. L. Ventola, "The Antibiotic Resistance Crisis: Part 2: Management Strategies and New Agents," *Pharmacy & Therapeutics* 40, no. 5 (May 2015): 344–52.

11. W. P. Bowe and A. C. Logan, "Acne Vulgaris, Probiotics, and the Gut-Brain-Skin Axis — Back to the Future?" *Gut Pathogens* 3, no. 1 (January 2011): 1; D. Sharma, M. M. Kober, and W. P. Bowe, "Anti-Aging Effects of Probiotics," *Journal of Drugs in Dermatology* 15, no. 1 (January 2016): 9–12.

12. S. Vandersee, et al., "Blue-Violet Light Irradiation Dose Dependently Decreases Carotenoids in Human Skin, Which Indicates the Generation of Free Radicals," *Oxidative Medicine and Cell Longevity* (2015): 579675.

13. P. Tullis, "The Man Who Can Map the Chemicals All Over Your Body," *Nature* 534, no. 7606 (June 2016).

Chapter 2: The New Science of Skin

1. A. Slominski, "A Nervous Breakdown in the Skin: Stress and the Epidermal Barrier," *Journal of Clinical Investigation* 117, no. 11 (November 2007): 3166–69; H. J. Hunter, S. E. Momen, and C. E. Kleyn, "The Impact of Psychosocial Stress on Healthy Skin," *Clinical and Experimental Dermatology* 40, no. 5 (July 2015) 540–46; M. Altemus, et al., "Stress-Induced Changes in Skin Barrier Function in Healthy Women," *Journal of Investigative Dermatology* 117, no. 2 (August 2001): 309–17.

2. W. P. Bowe and A. C. Logan, "Acne Vulgaris, Probiotics, and the Gut-Brain-Skin Axis — Back to the Future?" *Gut Pathogens* 3, no. 1 (January 2011): 1; D. Sharma, M. M. Kober, and W. P. Bowe, "Anti-Aging Effects of Probiotics," *Journal of Drugs in Dermatology* 15, no. 1 (January 2016): 9–12; W. Bowe, N. B. Patel, and A. C. Logan, "Acne Vulgaris, Probiotics, and the Gut-Brain-Skin Axis: From Anecdote to Translational Medicine," *Beneficial Microbes* 5, no. 2 (June 2014): 185–99.

3. J. H. Stokes and D. M. Pillsbury, "The Effect on the Skin of Emotional and Nervous States: Theoretical and Practical Consideration of a

Gastro-Intestinal Mechanism," *Archives of Dermatology and Syphilology* 22, no. 6 (1930): 962–93.

4. For a review of the field of psychodermatology, see G. E. Brown, et al., "Psychodermatology," *Advances in Psychosomatic Medicine* 34 (2015): 123–34.

5. "Stress and the Senstitive Gut," *Harvard Mental Health Letter,* August 2010, Harvard Health Publishing.

6. P. Hemarajata and J. Versalovic, "Effects of Probiotics on Gut Microbiota: Mechanisms of Intestinal Immunomodulation and Neuromodulation," *Therapeutic Advances in Gastroenterology* 6, no. 1 (January 2013): 39–51; C. H. Choi and S. K. Chang, "Alteration of Gut Microbiota and Efficacy of Probiotics in Functional Constipation," *Journal of Neurogastroenterology and Motility* 21, no. 1 (January 2015): 4–7; J. L. Sonnenburg and M. A. Fischbach, "Community Health Care: Therapeutic Opportunities in the Human Microbiome," *Science Translational Medicine* 3, no. 78 (April 2011).

7. R. Katta and S. P. Desai, "Diet and Dermatology: The Role of Dietary Intervention in Skin Disease," *Journal of Clinical and Aesthetic Dermatology* 7, no. 7 (July 2014): 46–51; R. Noordam, et al., "High Serum Glucose Levels Are Associated with a Higher Perceived Age," *Age* (Dordrecht) 35, no. 1 (February 2013): 189–95.

8. H. Zhang, et al., "Risk Factors for Sebaceous Gland Diseases and Their Relationship to Gastrointestinal Dysfunction in Han Adolescents," *Journal of Dermatology* 35, no. 9 (September 2008): 555–61.

9. J. Suez, et al., "Artificial Sweeteners Induce Glucose Intolerance by Altering the Gut Microbiota," *Nature* 514, no. 7521 (October 2014): 181–86; G. Fagherazzi, et al., "Consumption of Artificially and Sugar-Sweetened Beverages and Incident of Type 2 Diabetes in the Etude Epidemiologique Aupres des Femmes de la Mutuelle Generale de l'Education Nationale– European Prospective Investigation into Cancer and Nutrition Cohort," *American Journal of Clinical Nutrition* 97, no. 3 (2013): 517–23.

10. B. Chassaing, et al., "Dietary Emulsifiers Impact the Mouse Gut Microbiota Promoting Colitis and Metabolic Syndrome," *Nature* 519, no. 7541 (March 2015): 92–96; S. Reardon, "Food Preservatives Linked to Obesity and Gut Disease," Nature.com, February 25, 2015.

Chapter 3: Mind over Skin Matters

1. Hans Selye, "A Syndrome Produced by Diverse Nocuous Agents," *Nature* 138 (July 1936): 32; S. Szabo, Y. Tache, and A. Somogyi, "The Legacy of Hans Selye and the Origins of Stress Research: A Retrospec-

tive 75 Years after His Landmark Brief 'Letter' to the Editor of *Nature*," *Stress* 15, no. 5 (September 2012): 472–78; S. Szabo, et al., " 'Stress' Is 80 Years Old: From Hans Selye Original Paper in 1936 to Recent Advances in GI Ulceration," *Current Pharmaceutical Design* (June 2017).

2. "Walter Bradford Cannon (1871–1945), Harvard Physiologist," *Journal of the American Medical Association* 203, no. 12 (1968): 1063–65.

3. B. S. McEwen and E. Stellar, "Stress and the Individual: Mechanisms Leading to Disease," *Archives of Internal Medicine* 153, no. 18 (September 1993): 2093–2101.

4. S. Cohen, et al., "Chronic Stress, Glucocorticoid Receptor Resistance, Inflammation, and Disease Risk," *Proceedings of the National Academy of Sciences* 109, no. 16 (April 2012): 5995–99.

5. W. P. Bowe and A. C. Logan, "Acne Vulgaris, Probiotics, and the Gut-Brain-Skin Axis—Back to the Future?" *Gut Pathogens* 3, no. 1 (January 2011): 1.

6. R. L. O'Sullivan, G. Lipper, and E. A. Lerner, "The Neuro-Immuno-Cutaneous-Endocrine Network: Relationship of Mind and Skin," *Archives of Dermatology* 134, no. 11 (1998): 1431–35.

7. J. M. F. Hall, et al. "Psychological Stress and the Cutaneous Immune Response: Roles of the HPA Axis and the Sympathetic Nervous System in Atopic Dermatitis and Psoriasis," *Dermatology Research and Practice* 2012 (2012): 403908.

Chapter 4: Face Value

1. The figure was estimated by Allied Market Research and published in a report, available at https://www.alliedmarketresearch.com/press-release/skin-care-products-market.html.

2. E. Shklovskaya, et al., "Langerhans Cells Are Precommitted to Immune Tolerance Induction," *Proceedings of the National Academy of Sciences* 108, no. 44 (November 2011): 18049–54.

3. E. A. Grice and J. A. Segre, "The Skin Microbiome," *Nature Reviews: Microbiology* 9, no. 4 (April 2011): 244–53; M. Brandwein, D. Steinberg, and S. Meshner, "Microbial Biofilms and the Human Skin Microbiome," *NPJ Biofilms and Microbiomes* 2 (November 2016): 3.

4. T. Nakatsuji, et al., "The Microbiome Extends to Subepidermal Compartments of Normal Skin," *Nature Communications* 4 (2013): 1431.

5. P. L. Zeeuwen et al., "Microbiome Dynamics of Human Epidermis Following Skin Barrier Disruption," *Genome Biol.* 13, no. 11 (November 2012): R101.

6. E. Barnard, et al., "The Balance of Metagenomic Elements Shapes the Skin Microbiome in Acne and Health," *Scientific Reports* (2016).

7. "An Unbalanced Microbiome on the Face May Be Key to Acne Development," Medical Xpress, April 6, 2017, https://medicalxpress.com/news/2017-04-unbalanced-microbiome-key-acne.html.

8. Y. Belkaid and S. Tamoutounour, "The Influence of Skin Microorganisms on Cutaneous Immunity," *Nature Reviews: Immunology* 16, no. 6 (May 2016): 353–66; A. Azvolinsky, "Birth of the Skin Microbiome," *The Scientist,* November 17, 2015; T. C. Scharschmidt, et al., "A Wave of Regulatory T Cells into Neonatal Skin Mediates Tolerance to Commensal Microbes," *Immunity* 43, no. 5 (2015): 1011–21; H. J. Wu and E. Wu, "The Role of Gut Microbiota in Immune Homeostasis and Autoimmunity," *Gut Microbes* 3, no. 1 (January–February 2012): 4–14.

9. D. P. Strachan, "Hay Fever, Hygiene, and Household Size," *British Medical Journal* 299, no. 6710 (November 1989): 1259–60.

10. M. M. Stein, et al., "Innate Immunity and Asthma Risk in Amish and Hutterite Farm Children," *New England Journal of Medicine* 375, no. 5 (August 2016): 411–21.

11. Food and Drug Administration, "5 Things to Know About Triclosan" (April 8, 2010), at https://www.fda.gov/ForConsumers/Consumer Updates/ucm205999.htm.

Chapter 5: The Power in Going Pro

1. Review on Antimicrobial Resistance, *Antimicrobial Resistance: Tackling a Crisis for the Health and Wealth of Nations* (December 2014), at https://amr-review.org/sites/default/files/AMR%20Review%20Paper%20-%20 Tackling%20a%20crisis%20for%20the%20health%20and%20 wealth%20of%20nations_1.pdf.

2. M. G. Dominguez-Bello, et al., "Delivery Mode Shapes the Acquisition and Structure of the Initial Microbiota Across Multiple Body Habitats in Newborns," *Proceedings of the National Academy of Sciences* 107, no. 26 (June 2010): 11971–75; for a list of Dr. Dominguez-Bello's publications, go to her website at https://med.nyu.edu/faculty/maria-dominguez-bello.

3. I. Cho, et al., "Antibiotics in Early Life Alter the Murine Colonic Microbiome and Adiposity," *Nature* 488, no. 7413 (August 2012): 621–26.

4. L. M. Cox, et al., "Altering the Intestinal Microbiota During a Critical Developmental Window Has Lasting Metabolic Consequences," *Cell* 158, no. 4 (August 2014): 705–21.

5. M. M. Kober and W. P. Bowe, "The Effect of Probiotics on Immune Regulation, Acne, and Photoaging," *International Journal of Women's Dermatology* 2, no. 1 (April 2015): 85–89.

6. Because the volume of citations and studies covering the science of probiotics and skin health is too extensive to cover here, please refer to my 2015 paper (see note 5 above), which includes more than sixty references.

7. J. Benyacoub, et al., "Immune Modulation Property of *Lactobacillus paracasei* NCC2461 (ST11) Strain and Impact on Skin Defenses," *Beneficial Microbes* 5 (2014): 129–36.

8. B. S. Kang, et al., "Antimicrobial Activity of Enterocins from *Enterococcus faecalis* SL-5 Against *Propionibacterium acnes,* the Causative Agent in Acne Vulgaris, and Its Therapeutic Effect," *Journal of Microbiology* 41 (2009): 101–9.

9. N. Muizzuddin, et al., "Physiologic Effect of a Probiotic on the Skin," *Journal of Cosmetic Science* 63, no. 6 (2012): 385–95.

10. W. P. Bowe, et al., "Inhibition of *Propionibacterium acnes* by Bacteriocin-Like Inhibitory Substances (BLIS) Produced by *Streptococcus salivarius,*" *Journal of Drugs in Dermatology* 5, no. 9 (2006): 868–70.

11. J. R. Tagg, "Streptococcal Bacteriocin-Like Inhibitory Substances: Some Personal Insights into the Bacteriocin-Like Activities Produced by Streptococci Good and Bad," *Probiotics and Antimicrobial Proteins* 1, no. 1 (June 2009): 60–66.

12. W. P. Bowe, et al., "Inhibition of *Propionibacterium acnes* by Bacteriocin-Like Inhibitory Substances (BLIS) Produced by *Streptococcus salivarius,*" *Journal of Drugs in Dermatology* 5, no. 9 (2006): 868–70.

13. R. Gallo, et al., "Antimicrobials from Human Skin Commensal Bacteria Protect Against *Staphylococcus aureus* and Are Deficient in Atopic Dermatitis," *Science Translational Medicine* 9, no. 378 (February 2017).

14. A. Zipperer, et al., "Human Commensals Producing a Novel Antibiotic Impair Pathogen Colonization," *Nature* 535, no. 7613 (July 2016): 511–16.

15. K. Benson, et al., "Probiotic Metabolites from *Bacillus coagulans* GanedenBC30 Support Maturation of Antigen-Presenting Cells in Vitro," *World Journal of Gastroenterology* 18, no. 16 (2012): 1875–83; G.

Jensen, et al., "Ganeden BC30 Cell Wall and Metabolites: Anti-Inflammatory and Immune Modulating Effects in Vitro," *BMC Immunology* 11 (2010): 15.

16. M. Bruno-Barcena, et al., "Expression of a Heterologous Manganese Superoxide Dismutase Gene in Intestinal Lactobacilli Provides Protection Against Hydrogen Peroxide Toxicity," *Applied and Environmental Microbiology* 70, no. 8 (2004): 4702–10.

17. L. Di Marzio, et al., "Effect of the Lactic Acid Bacterium *Streptococcus thermophilus* on Ceramide Levels in Human Keratinocyte in Vitro and Stratum Corneum in Vivo," *Journal of Investigative Dermatology* 133 (1999): 98–106.

18. M. C. Peral, M. A. Martinez, and J. C. Valdez, "Bacteriotherapy with *Lactobacillus plantarum* in Burns," *International Wound Journal* 6, no. 1 (February 2009): 73–81.

19. S. Gordon, "Elie Metchnikoff: Father of Natural Immunity," *European Journal of Immunology* 38 (2008): 3257–64.

20. A. C. Ouwehand, S. Salminen, and E. Isolauri, "Probiotics: An Overview of Beneficial Effect," *Antonie Van Leeuwenhoek* 82 (2002): 279–89.

21. I. A. Rather, et al., "Probiotics and Atopic Dermatitis: An Overview," *Frontiers of Microbiology* 7 (April 2016): 507.

22. A. Gueniche, et al., "*Lactobacillus paracasei* CNCM I-2166 (ST11) Inhibits Substance P–Induced Skin Inflammation and Accelerates Skin Barrier Function Recovery in Vitro," *European Journal of Dermatology* 20, no. 6 (2010): 731–37; A. Gueniche, et al., "Randomised Double-Blind Placebo-Controlled Study of the Effect of *Lactobacillus paracasei* NCC 2461 on Skin Reactivity," *Beneficial Microbes* 5 (2014): 137–45.

23. I. A. Rather, et al., "Probiotics and Atopic Dermatitis: An Overview," *Frontiers of Microbiology* 7 (April 2016): 507; R. Frei, M. Akdis, and L. O'Mahony, "Prebiotics, Probiotics, Synbiotics, and the Immune System: Experimental Data and Clinical Evidence," *Current Opinion in Gastroenterology* 31, no. 2 (March 2015): 153–58.

24. H. M. Kim, et al., "Oral Administration of *Lactobacillus plantarum* HY7714 Protects Against Ultraviolet B–Induced Photoaging in Hairless Mice," *Journal of Microbiology and Biotechnology* 24 (2014): 1583–91.

25. C. Bouilly-Gauthier, et al. "Clinical Evidence of Benefits of a Dietary Supplement Containing Probiotic and Carotenoids on Ultraviolet-Induced Skin Damage," *British Journal of Dermatology* 163 (2010): 536–43.

26. Y. Ishii, et al., "Oral Administration of *Bifidobacterium breve* Attenuates UV-Induced Barrier Perturbation and Oxidative Stress in Hairless Mice Skin," *Archives of Dermatological Research* 305, no. 5 (2014): 467–73.

27. S. Sugimoto, et al. "Photoprotective Effects of *Bifidobacterium breve* Supplementation Against Skin Damage Induced by Ultraviolet Irradiation in Hairless Mice," *Photodermatology, Photoimmunology, and Photomedicine* 28 (2012): 312–19.

28. F. Marchetti, R. Capizzi, and A. Tulli, "Efficacy of Regulators of Intestinal Bacterial Flora in the Therapy of Acne Vulgaris," *La Clinica Terapeutica* 122 (1987): 339–43; L. A. Volkova, I. L. Khalif, and I. N. Kabanova, "Impact of Impaired Intestinal Microflora on the Course of Acne Vulgaris," *Klinicheskaia Meditsina* (2001): 7939–41; J. Kim, et al., "Dietary Effect of Lactoferrin-Enriched Fermented Milk on Skin Surface Lipid and Clinical Improvement in Acne Vulgaris," *Nutrition* 26 (2010): 902–9.

29. G. W. Jung, et al., "Prospective Randomized Open-Label Trial Comparing the Safety, Efficacy, and Tolerability of an Acne Treatment Regimen with and without a Probiotic Supplement in Subjects with Mild to Moderate Acne," *Journal of Cutaneous Medicine and Surgery* 17, no. 2 (2013): 114–22.

30. G. Jensen, et al., "Ganeden BC30 Cell Wall and Metabolites: Anti-Inflammatory and Immune Modulating Effects in Vitro," *BMC Immunology* 11 (2010): 15.

31. O. H. Mills, et al., "Addressing Free Radical Oxidation in Acne Vulgaris," *Journal of Clinical and Aesthetic Dermatology* 9, no. 1 (January 2016): 25–30.

Chapter 6: Feed Your Face

1. A. Pappas, A. Liakou, and C. C. Zouboulis, "Nutrition and Skin," *Reviews in Endocrine and Metabolic Disorders* 17, no. 3 (September 2016): 443–48.

2. R. Katta and S. P. Desai, "Diet and Dermatology: The Role of Dietary Intervention in Skin Disease," *Journal of Clinical and Aesthetic Dermatology* 7, no. 7 (July 2014): 46–51.

3. L. A. David, et al., "Diet Rapidly and Reproducibly Alters the Human Gut Microbiome," *Nature* 505, no. 7484 (January 2014): 559–63.

4. A. Manzel, et al., "Role of 'Western Diet' in Inflammatory Autoimmune Diseases," *Current Allergy and Asthma Reports* 14, no. 1 (January 2014): 404.

5. R. Katta and S. P. Desai, "Diet and Dermatology: The Role of Dietary Intervention in Skin Disease," *Journal of Clinical and Aesthetic Dermatology* 7, no. 7 (July 2014): 46–51.

6. W. P. Bowe, S. S. Joshi, and A. R. Shalita, "Diet and Acne," *Journal of the American Academy of Dermatology* 63, no. 1 (July 2010): 124–41.

7. S. N. Mahmood and W. P. Bowe, "Diet and Acne Update: Carbohydrates Emerge as the Main Culprit," *Journal of Drugs in Dermatology* 13, no. 4 (April 2014): 428–35.

8. D. Zeevi, et al., "Personalized Nutrition by Prediction of Glycemic Responses," *Cell* 163, no. 5 (2015): 1079–94.

9. United States Department of Agriculture Economic Research Service, "Food Availability and Consumption," 2016, at https://www.ers.usda .gov/data-products/ag-and-food-statistics-charting-the-essentials/ food-availability-and-consumption/.

10. Dr. Robert Lustig, of the University of California at San Francisco, has been sounding the alarm about sugars, particularly processed fructose, for many years now, as detailed in numerous scientific publications and in his book *Fat Chance: Beating the Odds Against Sugar, Processed Food, Obesity, and Disease* (New York: Hudson Street Press, 2012).

11. Q. Zhang, et al., "A Perspective on the Maillard Reaction and the Analysis of Protein Glycation by Mass Spectrometry: Probing the Pathogenesis of Chronic Disease," *Journal of Proteome Research* 8 (2009): 754–69.

12. J. Uribarri, et al., "Diet-Derived Advanced Glycation End Products Are Major Contributors to the Body's AGE Pool and Induce Inflammation in Healthy Subjects," *Annals of the New York Academy of Sciences* 1043 (2005): 461–66; M. Negrean, et al., "Effects of Low- and High-Advanced Glycation Endproduct Meals on Macro- and Microvascular Endothelial Function and Oxidative Stress in Patients with Type 2 Diabetes Mellitus," *American Journal of Clinical Nutrition* 85 (2007): 1236–43.

13. E. Baye, et al., "Effect of Dietary Advanced Glycation End Products on Inflammation and Cardiovascular Risks in Healthy Overweight Adults: A Randomised Crossover Trial," *Scientific Reports* 7, no. 1 (June 2017): 4123.

14. T. Goldberg, et al., "Advanced Glycoxidation End Products in Commonly Consumed Foods," *Journal of the American Dietetic Association* 104 (2004): 1287–91; J. Uribarri, et al., "Advanced Glycation End Products in Foods and a Practical Guide to Their Reduction in the Diet," *Journal of the American Dietetic Association* 110 (2010): 911–16.

15. M. Yaar and B. A. Gilchrest, "Photoageing: Mechanism, Prevention and Therapy," *British Journal of Dermatology* 157, no. 5 (2007): 874–87.

16. A. Vojdani, "A Potential Link between Environmental Triggers and Autoimmunity," *Autoimmune Diseases* 2014 (2014): 437231.

17. C. Pontes Tde, et al., "Incidence of Acne Vulgaris in Young Adult Users of Protein-Calorie Supplements in the City of João Pessoa, PB," *Anais brasileiros de ginecologia* 88, no. 6 (November–December 2013): 907–12; C. L. LaRosa, et al., "Consumption of Dairy in Teenagers with and without Acne," *Journal of the American Academy of Dermatology* 75, no. 2 (August 2016): 318–22.

18. R. Katta and D. N. Brown, "Diet and Skin Cancer: The Potential Role of Dietary Antioxidants in Nonmelanoma Skin Cancer Prevention," *Journal of Skin Cancer* (2015).

19. M. Furue, et al., "Antioxidants for Healthy Skin: The Emerging Role of Aryl Hydrocarbon Receptors and Nuclear Factor-Erythroid 2-Related Factor-2," *Nutrients* 9, no. 3 (March 2017); S. K. Schagen, et al., "Discovering the Link between Nutrition and Skin Aging," *Dermato-Endocrinology* 4, no. 3 (July 2012): 298–307.

20. K. Wertz, et al., "Beta-Carotene Inhibits UVA-Induced Matrix Metalloprotease 1 and 10 Expression in Keratinocytes by a Singlet Oxygen-Dependent Mechanism," *Free Radical Biology and Medicine* 37, no. 5 (September 2004): 654–70.

21. O. H. Mills, et al., "Addressing Free Radical Oxidation in Acne Vulgaris," *Journal of Clinical and Aesthetic Dermatology* 9, no. 1 (January 2016): 25–30.

22. For a great overview of fatty acids and skin health, go to the Micronutrient Information Center at Oregon State University's Linus Pauling Institute and read "Essential Fatty Acids and Skin Health," at http://lpi .oregonstate.edu/mic/health-disease/skin-health/essential-fatty-acids.

23. G. M. Balbás, M. S. Regaña, and P. U. Millet, "Study on the Use of Omega-3 Fatty Acids as a Therapeutic Supplement in Treatment of Psoriasis," *Clinical, Cosmetic, and Investigational Dermatology* 4 (2011): 73–77.

Chapter 7: Take Time to Recover

1. A. Safdar, et al., "Endurance Exercise Rescues Progeroid Aging and Induces Systemic Mitochondrial Rejuvenation in MTDNA Mutator Mice," *Proceedings of the National Academy of Sciences* 108, no. 10 (March 2011): 4135–40.

2. J. D. Crane, et al., "Exercise-Stimulated Interleukin-15 Is Controlled by AMPK and Regulates Skin Metabolism and Aging," *Aging Cell* 14, no. 4 (August 2015): 625–34.

3. The volume of literature on the benefits of exercise could fill a library. You can easily check out a multitude of studies online just by googling "benefits of exercise" or going to the websites of organizations such as the Mayo Clinic (www.MayoClinic.org) and Harvard Health Publishing (www.Health.Harvard.edu).

4. N. Owen, et al., "Too Much Sitting: The Population Health Science of Sedentary Behavior," *Exercise and Sport Sciences Reviews* 38, no. 3 (July 2010): 105–13.

5. For more about the relaxation response, including one of Dr. Benson's step-by-step guides to triggering it, go to www.RelaxationResponse .org. You can also visit the Benson-Henry Institute at www.Benson HenryInstitute.org.

6. S. W. Lazar, et al., "Meditation Experience Is Associated with Increased Cortical Thickness," *Neuroreport* 16, no. 17 (November 28, 2005): 1893–97.

7. I. Buric, et al., "What Is the Molecular Signature of Mind–Body Interventions? A Systematic Review of Gene Expression Changes Induced by Meditation and Related Practices," *Frontiers in Immunology* 8 (June 2017): 670.

8. For a full list of useful references and resources on the power of sleep, visit the National Sleep Foundation at https://SleepFoundation.org/.

9. K. Spiegel, et al., "Brief Communication: Sleep Curtailment in Healthy Young Men Is Associated with Decreased Leptin Levels, Elevated Ghrelin Levels, and Increased Hunger and Appetite," *Annals of Internal Medicine* 141, no. 11 (December 7, 2004): 846–50.

10. C. A. Thaiss, et al., "Microbiota Diurnal Rhythmicity Programs Host Transcriptome Oscillations," *Cell* (December 2016).

11. M. R. Irwin, et al., "Sleep Loss Activates Cellular Inflammatory Signaling," *Biological Psychiatry* 64, no. 6 (September 2008): 538–40.

12. A. M. Chang, et al., "Evening Use of Light-Emitting Ereaders Negatively Affects Sleep, Circadian Timing, and Next-Morning Alertness," *Proceedings of the National Academy of Sciences* 112, no. 4 (January 2015): 1232–37.

13. S. Panda, et al., "Time-Restricted Feeding Is a Preventative and Therapeutic Intervention Against Diverse Nutritional Challenges," *Cell Metabolism* 20, no. 6 (2014): 991–1005; S. Panda, et al., "Diet and Feed-

ing Pattern Affect the Diurnal Dynamics of the Gut Microbiome," *Cell Metabolism* 20, no. 6 (2014): 1006–17.

Chapter 8: Handle with Care

1. M. Randhawa, et al., "Daily Use of a Facial Broad-Spectrum Sunscreen Over One Year Significantly Improves Clinical Evaluation of Photoaging," *Dermatologic Surgery* 42, no. 12 (December 2016): 1354–61.
2. M. C. Aust, et al., "Percutaneous Collagen Induction-Regeneration in Place of Cicatrisation?" *Journal of Plastic, Reconstructive, and Aesthetic Surgery* 64, no. 1 (January 2011): 97–107. doi: 10.1016/j.bjps.2010.03.038. Epub April 21, 2010.
3. For an online resource for checking medications and their potential side effects on skin, go to www.RxList.com.

Chapter 9: Supercharge Your Skin

1. S. K. Schagen, et al., "Discovering the Link between Nutrition and Skin Aging," *Dermato-Endocrinology* 4, no. 3 (July 2012): 298–307; For an overview of vitamin E and its role in skin health, go to the Micronutrient Information Center at Oregon State University's Linus Pauling Institute and read "Vitamin E and Skin Health," at http://lpi.oregon state.edu/mic/health-disease/skin-health/vitamin-E.
2. For an overview of vitamin C and its role in skin health, go to the Micronutrient Information Center at Oregon State University's Linus Pauling Institute and read "Vitamin C and Skin Health," at http://lpi .oregonstate.edu/mic/health-disease/skin-health/vitamin-C.
3. For an overview of vitamin D and its role in skin health, go to the Micronutrient Information Center at Oregon State University's Linus Pauling Institute and read "Vitamin C and Skin Health," at http://lpi .oregonstate.edu/mic/health-disease/skin-health/vitamin-D.
4. J. F. Scott, et al., "Oral Vitamin D Rapidly Attenuates Inflammation from Sunburn: An Interventional Study," *Journal of Investigative Dermatology* (May 2017).
5. For more about Heliocare, go to http://www.Heliocare.com/.

Index

acne
  antioxidants in treating, 131
  cell phones and, 183
  diet's role in, 10, 26–27, 57, 59,
    118–19, 126
  evening primrose oil in, 230
  masks for, 244–45, 246
  oral antibiotics in treating,
    106–7, 191–92
  oral probiotics in treating, 106–7
  retinoids in treating, 175, 177
  role of *P. acnes* in, 85–86, 97, 100
  statistics on, 12, 22
  stress and, 64
  substance P and, 75
  topical antibiotics in treating,
    100–101, 177–78, 191, 226
  topical probiotics in treating, 98,
    171, 173
  zinc in treating, 190
adrenal glands, 38
adrenaline, 38, 68, 151
advanced glycation end products
    (AGEs), 123–24, 125
aging of skin, 82, 145–46, 182
  accelerated, quiz on risk factors
    for, 45–47
  discoloration and, 83–84
exercise and, 144–45
glycation-related, 124–25
premature, 168–70, 173, 244–45
probiotics for, 102–3, 244–45
AHAs (alpha hydroxy acids),
    168–69, 170, 175
air pollution, 36
ALA (alpha-linolenic acid), 133
alcohol, 138, 157, 216, 224–25
allergic rhinitis, 89
allergies, 88–89
allostasis, 68
allostatic load, 68
almond butter, 219
almond flour, 237
almond milk, 61, 127, 139, 215,
    234, 235, 236
almonds, 141
alpha hydroxy acids (AHAs),
    168–69, 170, 175
alpha-linolenic acid (ALA), 133
American Academy of
    Dermatology, 9–10, 171
antibiotic resistance, 12–13, 39–40,
    92, 100–101
antibiotics, 3
  in acne treatment, 100–101,
    106–7, 177–78, 191–92, 226

antibiotics *(cont.)*
  discovery of, 91–92, 101
  effect of frequent use in
    children, 88
  obesity and, 36, 93–94
  in rosacea treatment, 94, 192
antimicrobial peptides, 87, 96, 99
antimicrobials, avoiding, 92
antioxidant serums, 165–66,
    226–27, 228
antioxidants
  Cranberry-Apple Antioxidant
    Face Mask, 231
  dietary, benefits of, 129–32,
    139–40, 190
  in topical skin-care products,
    159, 182
apples, 139, 216, 231
artificial sweeteners, 59, 61, 122,
    123, 138, 208, 215
asparagus, 120, 140, 242–43
asthma, 89
atopic dermatitis. *See* eczema
atopic march, 89
autoimmune diseases, 22, 31, 88
autoimmunity, development of, 87
avocado oil, 213
avocados, 139, 212, 216, 217
  Avocado Mousse, 218, 243
  Coconut-Oil Mask with
    Avocado, 247
  Honey Avocado Yogurt Mask,
    174
  Rich Avocado Truffles, 219, 244
  Savory Avo-Yogurt Dip, 242

Bacillus coagulans, 102, 103, 107,
    173, 195
bacteria

body's symbiotic relationship
    with, 32–33
  global toll of deaths related to, 91
  healthy, strengthening, 39–42
  resistant to antibiotics, 12–13,
    39–40
  in small intestinal bacterial
    overgrowth (SIBO), 55–59, 64
  species in skin, 7, 85
  See also probiotics
Balsamic Vinaigrette, 238
bananas, 139, 219
  Chocolate Banana Mousse, 218,
    243
  Strawberry Banana Overnight
    Oats, 219, 236
Barnard, Emma, 85, 86
basil, 217, 240–41
beans, 141
beef, organic, 141
bell peppers
  Big Hearty Salad, 237–38
  Hearty Vegetable Dinner
    Scramble, 239–40
  Pineapple Chicken Skewers, 217,
    240–41
Benson, Herbert, 150
benzoyl peroxide, 164, 177–78, 226
berries, 139, 216
  Bowe Glow Berry Smoothie,
    217, 219, 234–35
  Dandelion-Green Smoothie,
    219, 235
  See also specific berries
beta-carotene, 130
beta hydroxy acids (BHAs), 169,
    170, 175
beverages
  to avoid, 137–38, 208, 215

recipes for, 234–36
in week 1 of program, 207–8,
 210, 214–16
See also specific beverages
BHAs (beta hydroxy acids), 169,
 170, 175
Bifidobacterium breve, 105, 195
Bifidobacterium genera, 104,
 105–6, 195
biotin, 196
blackberries, 236
Blaser, Martin, 93–94
blood sugar levels, 35, 115, 119, 128.
 See also insulin levels
blood vessels, 80, 81, 82, 146
body bar/wash, 226, 227–28
Bowe, Whitney, 10–11, 84, 95
 decision to become a doctor,
  3–4, 160–61
 illness during childhood, 3
 patented acne treatment
  coinvented by, 8
 skin of, 77–78
 website of, 163
brain
 development of, 37, 53
 relaxation response and, 150
 See also gut-brain-skin
  relationship; mind-body
  relationship
branzino, 140–41, 218
breakfast, 128–29, 217–19, 236–37
broccoli, 120, 237–38, 242–43
bubonic plague, 91
butter, 213

C. diff, 3, 107
caffeine, 157, 215, 224–25
calcium, 189, 206

calories in diet, 35, 115, 121, 125,
 213
cancer, skin, 12, 22, 78, 129, 163, 187
Cannon, Walter Bradford, 67
carbohydrates, 110, 118–19, 120,
 208, 212
cardiorespiratory fitness, 148
carotenoids, 105, 130, 139, 140
carrots, 130, 140
casein, 126
cashews, 141
catechins, 132
cauliflower, 242–43
cell phones, 183
central nervous system, 36–37, 54,
 74, 75
ceramides, 103, 172, 182
Chang, Anne-Marie, 157
cheese, 127, 128, 209
chemical peels, 170
chia seeds, 141, 236
chicken, 141, 219
 Big Hearty Salad, 237–38
 Broiled Honey-Orange-Lemon
  Chicken, 219, 241
 Decadent Salad with Spinach,
  Crushed Walnuts, Sliced
  Strawberries, and, 219, 238
 Pineapple Chicken Skewers, 217,
  240–41
Chilean sea bass, 219
chocolate, 217, 220
 Chocolate Banana Mousse, 218,
  243
 Rich Avocado Truffles, 219, 244
cilantro, 242
cinnamon, 114, 142, 235
circadian rhythms, 154–55, 157, 224
cleanliness, excessive, 88–89

clindamycin, 177, 226

Clostridium difficile, 3, 107

coconut milk, 61, 127, 139, 236

coconut oil, 213–14, 230

    Coconut-Oil Mask with
      Avocado, 247

    Oatmeal Coconut-Oil Power
      Mask, 246

    Probiotic Power Mask, 245

coffee, 130, 138, 213, 215, 245

collagen, 71–72, 74, 76, 131, 175,
    177, 190

collagen induction therapy. *See*
    microneedling

commensal symbiosis, 29

condiments, 209

Consumer Reports, 168

ConsumerLab, 196

copper, 190–91, 206

corticotropin-releasing hormone
    (CRH), 71, 74–75

cortisol, 37, 38, 68, 71, 72, 151,
    154–55

Cranberry-Apple Antioxidant Face
    Mask, 231

cranial nerves, 54

CRH. *See* corticotropin-releasing
    hormone (CRH)

Crohn's disease, 59

cucumbers, 214, 236, 237–38

dairy products, 10, 125–29, 138–39,
    208. *See also specific dairy
    products*

Dandelion-Green Smoothie, 219,
    235

dark chocolate, 217, 219, 220, 244

deep breathing, 151–52, 220, 223

Demodex, 97

dermatology, 9–11

dermis, 81, 145

dessert, 217–20, 243–44

Detox Water, 214, 236

DHA (docosahexaenoic acid),
    133, 196

diet

    high-whey, 26–27

    skin quality and, 9–11, 48–49, 60

    small intestinal bacterial
      overgrowth (SIBO) and,
      55–59, 60

    super-low-carb, 212

diet iced tea, 137

diet soft drinks, 59

dietary protocol, 113–42

    antioxidants in, 129–32

    beverages in, 207–8, 210, 214–16

    dairy products in, 125–29

    grocery shopping for, 138–42,
      210–12

    low-glycemic, whole, and
      unprocessed foods in, 118–25,
      207–9

    omega-3s vs. omega-6s in,
      132–34, 209, 212–13

    overview of, 113–17

    prebiotics and probiotics in,
      134–36, 209

    sample menu for, 217–20

dill, 217, 240–41

dinner, 217–20, 239–41

Dip, Savory Avo-Yogurt, 242

discoloration, skin, 177, 178–79, 187

DNA shotgun sequencing analysis, 86

docosahexaenoic acid (DHA), 133,
    196

Dominguez-Bello, Maria Gloria, 93

Dorrestein, Pieter, 44

double cleansing, 229
dry skin, mask for, 247
dull skin, mask for, 244–45
dysbiosis, 29

earbuds, 183
eczema, 22, 89
  inflammation in, 52
  masks for, 244–45, 246
  stress and, 64
  treating, 101–2, 192, 230
eggs, 128–29, 139, 216, 217, 219,
  239–40
eicosapentaenoic acid (EPA), 133, 196
elastin, 74, 76, 190
emulsifiers, 60
endorphins, 37, 74
enteric nervous system, 54
Enterococcus faecalis, 98, 103, 173
EPA (eicosapentaenoic acid), 133, 196
epidermis, 82–84, 145, 189
erythromycin, 177, 226
evening primrose oil, 230
exercise, 49, 143–49, 220–23
exfoliating, 24–25, 49, 168–70, 171,
  228, 245
extra-virgin olive oil, 142, 213, 214
eye cream, 230

facial cleansers, daily, 48, 49, 226, 228
fats, dietary, 132–34, 208–9, 212–13
FDA (Food and Drug
  Administration), 90, 92, 168,
  194
fermentation, 134–35
fermented products, 104, 127,
  134–35, 138–39, 193
fiber, prolonged stress and diets low
  in, 55–59, 60

fibroblasts, 81–82, 186–87, 190
fight-or-flight response, 37, 38, 67, 71
figs, 237
fine lines, 177, 181
fish, 237–38. *See also specific fish*
Fleming, Alexander, 101
food
  choices as fundamental to
    immune system health, 33
  as data for DNA and
    microbiome, 114–15
  gluten-free, 210
  nutrition labels for, 210–11
  purchasing, 138–42, 211–12
  in week 1 of program, 207–10
  See also diet
Food and Drug Administration
  (FDA), 90, 92, 168, 194
food journaling, 116, 212
free radicals, 72, 105–6, 107, 124,
  125, 131, 165
fructose, 121–22
fruit, 130–31, 139–40, 212. *See also
  specific fruit*
fungi, 7, 85, 99

(GAGs). *See* glycosaminoglycans
  (GAGs)
Gallo, Richard, 101
GALT (gut-associated lymphoid
  tissue), 33
garlic
  Balsamic Vinaigrette, 238
  Hearty Roasted Veggie Mix,
    220, 242–43
  Pineapple Chicken Skewers, 217,
    240–41
general adaptation syndrome, 66
ghee, 213

ghrelin, 154
glucose, 121
glutathione peroxidase, 191
gluten-free food, 210
glycation end products, 121–22
glycation-related aging, 123–25
glycemic index, 119–23, 232
glycemic load, 115, 120
glycolic acids, 168–69, 170, 175, 228
glycosaminoglycans (GAGs), 81
Golden Milk, 216, 219, 235
Goldin, Barry, 104–5
Google Calendar, 232
Gorbach, Sherwood, 104–5
Gordon, Jeffrey, 34
Gordon Lab, 36
grains, low-glycemic-index, 209
grapefruit, 139
Greek-style yogurt, 138, 216, 218, 242, 245
Green Tea and Honey Power Mask for Combating Redness, 246
grocery list, 138–42, 232
gut-associated lymphoid tissue (GALT), 33
gut-brain-skin relationship, 5, 6, 8, 28–33, 48–50, 52–55

hair, thinning, 196–97
hair follicles, 81
hand-free devices, 183
hand sanitizers, 90, 226
hay fever, 89
hazelnuts, 141
heliocare, 188–89, 206
herbs, 209
high-fructose corn syrup, 121, 125
high-glycemic foods, 62, 115, 118, 119

high-whey diets, adult acne and, 26–27
Hippocrates, 28–29
histamines, 74
honey
    Broiled Honey-Orange-Lemon Chicken, 219, 241
    Green Tea and Honey Power Mask, 246
    Honey Avocado Yogurt Mask, 174
    Probiotic Power Mask with Jojoba Oil and Honey, 245
    Probiotic Power Mask with Turmeric and Honey, 244–45
hormones
    circadian rhythms and, 154
    disturbances in, skin and, 70, 82
    function of, 69
    stress, 38, 66, 71, 72, 73–76, 151
    See also specific hormones
HPA (hypothalamic-pituitary-adrenal) axis, 70–76
Human Genome Project, 33
human microbiome, 6–7, 29–30, 45–47, 93, 114–15. *See also specific microbiomes*
hyaluronic acid, 81, 230
hydroquinone, 179
hygiene hypothesis, 88–89
hyperpigmentation, 178–79
hypothalamic-pituitary-adrenal (HPA) axis, 70–76
hypothalamus, 70–71, 158

ice cream, 208
IFOS (International Fish Oil Standards Program), 196
immune system, 31, 33, 78, 87, 88–89, 93

immunity, sleep deprivation and, 155–56
inflammation, 32, 49
  in acne, 131
  evening primrose oil in reducing, 230
  mask for, 246
  probiotics in reducing, 98, 104, 192–93
  sleep deprivation and, 155–56
  in small intestinal bacterial overgrowth (SIBO), 56–57, 64
  during stress, 65, 72, 73–74, 75
  Western diet and, 115, 116–17
inflammatory bowel disease, 59
inflammatory response, 31
infrared light, 42
insomnia, 156–59
insulin levels, 115, 119, 121, 123, 126
International Fish Oil Standards Program (IFOS), 196
intestinal bacteria
  antibiotics' impact on, 93–94
  artificial sweeteners and, 138
  gut permeability and, 51–52
  in SIBO, 55–59, 60, 64
intestinal flora, 29, 30–31, 52–55, 61
intestinal microbes, 13, 28–32, 34–35, 50, 155
intestinal microbiome
  amount of time to change health and function of, 116
  functions of, 86, 87
  imbalance and gut dysfunction, 59, 70
  of infants, 87
  link between metabolism and, 31, 34–35, 50

probiotics' ability to help recolonize, 13
intestinal wall, 51, 78
iron, 196, 207

jojoba oil, 245
Journal of Dermatology, 58
Journal of Skin Cancer, 129

kale, 114, 140, 187
kefir, 99, 127, 138, 193, 209
keratinocytes, 82–83
kimchi, 104, 134, 135, 193, 209
Knight, Rob, 34
Knight Lab, 36
Kober, Mary-Margaret, 95
kombucha, 104, 138, 215–16

labels for food, nutrition, 210–11
lactic acid fermentation, 135
Lactobacillus acidophilus, 135
Lactobacillus bulgaricus, 171
Lactobacillus genera, 104–5, 195
Lactobacillus johnsonii, 105
Lactobacillus paracasei, 98, 104, 173, 195
Lactobacillus plantarum, 98, 103, 105, 173, 195
Lactobacillus rhamnosus GG, 104–5
Langerhans cells, 83, 105
leafy greens, 42, 114, 119, 140, 190–91
"leaky gut," 51, 57, 58
"leaky skin," 51–52
legumes, 141
lemons, 140
  Broiled Honey-Orange-Lemon Chicken, 219, 241
  Detox Water, 214, 236
  Pineapple Chicken Skewers, 217, 240–41

lentigo, 178
leptin, 154
lifestyle habits, 24–27, 113
limes, 140, 242
linoleic acid, 230
Logan, Alan C., 57
low-glycemic foods, 62, 115, 119, 209
lunch, 217–19, 237–39
lycopene, 130, 131–32, 140
lymph vessels, 80, 81
lymphocytes, 33, 84–85

macadamia nuts, 141
Maillard, Louis Camille, 123
makeup, using, 228–29
makeup remover, recipe for, 229
mango, 140
Margolis, David, 8, 99, 100
masks, 174, 226, 230–31, 244–47
mast cells, 74–75
Mayo Clinic, 12
McEwen, Bruce, 68
meals, 213
    planning, 211, 232
    recipes for, 234–44
    sample menu for, 217–20
Mechnikov, Elie, 103–4
meditation, 149–52, 205, 223–24,
    231, 232
melanin, 83
melanocytes, 83–84, 187
melanoma, 187
melasma, 178
melatonin, 155
mental health disorders, 53
menu for a week, sample, 217–20
metabolism, 31, 34–35, 50, 123
methicillin-resistant *Staphylococcus
    aureus* (MRSA), 101

microbial profile, 32–33, 43–44,
    85–86, 88
microbiome, 6, 29. *See also* human
    microbiome; skin microbiome
microbiome sequencing, 43–44,
    85–86
microbiota, 29
microneedling, 179–80, 181
milk
    alternative, 127, 139
    cows', 125–26, 127, 208, 209,
        213, 215, 219
    Golden Milk, 216, 219
mind-body relationship
    relaxation response and, 150–51,
        159, 223–24
    stress in, 65–76
    in week 2 of program, 220–25
mitochondria, 145–46
moisturizers, 227, 228, 230
MRSA. *See* methicillin-resistant
    Staphylococcus aureus (MRSA)
multivitamins, 130, 186, 189–90, 206
mushrooms, 239–40, 242–43
mutualistic symbiosis, 29, 32
MyFitnessPal app, 212, 232

nails, brittle, 196–97
nervous system, 36–37, 53–54, 74,
    75, 151
neurons, 54
neuropeptides, 75
NICE (neuro-immuno-cutaneous-
    endocrine) network, 73
non-rapid eye movement
    (NREM), 155
Nothias-Scaglia, Louis-Felix, 43–44
NREM (non-rapid eye movement),
    155

NSF International, 196
nutmeg, 247
nutrition labels for food, 210–11
nuts, 141, 212, 216

oatmeal, 142, 218
oats, 142, 218, 219, 236, 246
obesity, 34–35, 36, 93–94, 122
oil glands. *See* sebaceous glands
olive oil, extra-virgin, 142, 213, 214
omega-3 fatty acids, 132–34, 139,
   140–41, 196, 207, 209
omega-6 fatty acids, 133–34, 209
omega-9 fatty acids, 134
onions
   Hearty Roasted Veggie Mix,
      220, 242–43
   Hearty Vegetable Dinner
      Scramble, 239–40
   Pineapple Chicken Skewers, 217,
      240–41
   Savory Avo-Yogurt Dip, 242
oranges, 139, 219, 241
overcleansing, 24–25, 26
oxidation, 72

Pancakes, Bowe Glow, 219, 237
Panda, Satchidananda, 158
parasitic symbiosis, 29
parasympathetic nervous system,
   151
Pasteur, Louis, 135
peanut butter, 213
peanuts, 141, 213
peas, 141
peptides, 75, 182, 230
phospholipid bilayer, 132
photoaging, 42
photosensitivity, 130

PIH (postinflammatory
   hyperpigmentation), 178
Pilates, 222, 223
Pillsbury, Donald M., 52, 56, 58
pineal gland, 155
Pineapple Chicken Skewers, 217,
   240–41
pistachios, 141, 218
pollution, 36
polyphenols, 132, 142
Polypodium leucotomos, 188
polyunsaturated fats, 132–33
pork, 141
postbiotics, 96, 172
postinflammatory
   hyperpigmentation (PIH),
   178
prebiotics, 41–42, 136, 172, 209
probiotics, 13, 41–42, 91–107
   definition of, 41
   in foods and beverages, 127, 128,
      134–36, 138, 193, 209
   oral, 25–26, 42, 52, 57, 104–7,
      192–96, 206, 226
   topical, 41–42, 95–103, 171–74,
      226, 244–45
processed foods, 55, 60, 118, 120,
   132, 208, 213
Propionibacterium acnes, 85–86, 97,
   99, 100
protein, 71–72, 74, 209
psoriasis, 22, 43, 64, 134, 192, 230,
   245
psychodermatology
   (psychocutaneous medicine),
   53, 150
pumpkin seeds, 141

quinoa, 217, 218, 238–39

rapid eye movement (REM), 155
relaxation response, 150–51, 159,
    223–24
Relaxation Response, The (Benson),
    150
REM (rapid eye movement), 155
restaurants, 232
resveratrol, 138
retinoids, 170, 174–77, 181
retinol, 169, 175, 176, 227, 230
rooibos tea, 216
rosacea, 22, 52
    masks for, 244–45, 246
    role of *Demodex* in, 97
    statistics on, 22
    during stress, 64
    treatment of, 94, 98–99, 173,
        192, 230
    triggers in, 13
rosemary, 238, 242–43

salad dressing, 211, 238
salads, 217, 218, 219, 237–38
salicylic acid, 181
salmon, 141, 217, 218, 238–39
SALT (skin-associated lymphoid
    tissue), 33, 84–85
sanitizers, hand, 90, 226
sardines, 140–41
sauerkraut, 134, 135, 209
sebaceous glands, 81
seeds, 141
selenium, chelated, 191, 206
Selye, Hans, 66–67
serotonin, 30–31, 54
serums, antioxidant, 165–66,
    226–27, 228, 230
Shirota, Minoru, 104
shopping, grocery, 138–42, 210–11

SIBO (small intestinal bacterial
    overgrowth), 55–59, 64
skim milk, 61, 126
skin
    anatomy of, 79–84
    development of, 36–37, 53
    functions of, 51
    gut–brain–skin relationship, 5, 6,
        8, 28–33, 48–50, 52–55
    healthy, pH of, 103
    myths about, 42–43
    overcleansing, 24–26
    as a reflection of overall health, 5,
        23, 42–43
    stress response triggered by,
        37–38, 73–76
skin-associated lymphoid tissue
    (SALT), 33, 84–85
skin cancer, 12, 22, 78, 129, 163, 187
skin-care brands, 163, 164
skin-care routine, 78, 161–84,
    225–31
    adding latest trends into, 179–80
    daily commitment to, 164–65
    for discoloration, 178–79
    in evening, 229–31
    exfoliation in, 168–70
    in morning, 227–29
    purchasing products for, 226–27
    retinoids in, 174–77
    skin-prep checklist for, 225–27
    Sugar Scrub recipe for, 171
    sun protection in, 166–68
    through the decades, 180–83
    topical probiotics in, 171–74, 226
skin color, 83–84
skin discoloration, 177, 178–79, 187
skin disorders, quiz on risk factors
    for, 45–47

skin flora, 29, 85

skin microbiome, 84–90, 161–64, 171–72

skyr, 139

sleep, 31, 155–59, 224–25, 231–32

sleep apnea, 158

sleep deprivation, 152–54, 155–56

sleep study, 158

small intestinal bacterial overgrowth (SIBO), 55–59, 64

smoking, 82, 124

smoothies, 217, 219, 234–35

snacks, 211, 213, 216–17, 220, 242–43

soft drinks, diet, 59

spices, 209

spinach, 114, 140, 219, 238, 239–40

squash, 140

Staphylococcus aureus, 101–2

Staphylococcus epidermidis, 101

Staphylococcus hominis, 101

Staphylococcus lugdunensis, 102

Stellar, Eliot, 68

stevia, 59

Stokes, John H., 52, 56, 58

Strachan, David, 88

stratum corneum, 83, 145

strawberries, 219, 236, 238

Strawberry Banana Overnight Oats, 219, 236

Streptococcus salivarius, 99–100, 101, 173

Streptococcus thermophilus, 103

stress, 65–69

biology of, 69–76

as contributing to body's chaos and angry skin, 49, 50, 52–59, 60, 64, 65, 143

definition of, 65, 66–67

managing, 55, 147, 150–52, 159, 223–24

subcategories of, 68

stress hormones, 38, 66, 71, 72, 73–76, 151

stress response, 37–38

stressors, 74–75

substance P, 75–76, 98

sugar

acne and, 10, 118–19, 126

artificial, 59, 61, 122, 123, 138, 208, 215

changes to the body from, 118–19, 120–22

elimination of, 120–21

other names for, 121, 122

refined, 121, 208

stimulation of glycation, 125

sugar alcohols, 59

Sugar Scrub recipe, 171

sun protection, rules for, 166–68

sunburn, mask for, 245

sunflower seeds, 141

sunscreens, 42, 165, 166–68, 181, 227, 228

supernatants, 96

supplements, recommendations on, 185–97, 205–7

sweat glands, 80

sweet addiction, 116

sweet potatoes, 130

sweeteners

artificial, 59, 61, 123, 138, 208, 215

natural, 209

symbiotic relationships, 29, 32

Tagg, John, 100

Tarnopolsky, Mark, 145, 146

tea, 104, 137, 138, 215–16, 246

tolerance, development of, 87
tomatoes
    lycopene in, 130, 131, 140
    recipes with, 237–38, 242
trace minerals, 189–91, 206
trans fats, 132
triclosan, 90
trout, 140–41
Truffles, Rich Avocado, 219, 244
turkey, 141, 218
turmeric, 142, 244–45

ulcerative colitis, 59
United Nations, 92
unprocessed foods, 118, 120,
    232, 234
US Pharmacopeial Convention
    (USP), 196
UV rays
    age and, 83–84
    protection from, 102, 105–6,
        165, 166–67, 188–89
    skin damage from, 42, 82

vagus nerve, 54
van Leeuwenhoek, Anton, 91, 92
vegetable oils, 133
vegetables
    antioxidants in, 130–31, 140, 212
    recipes with, 218, 220, 238–40,
        242–43
    roasted, 214, 217, 239, 242–43
    as snacks, 216
    See also specific vegetables
viruses, 7, 99

visible light, threatening sources
    of, 42
vitamin A, 130, 135, 140, 175, 206
vitamin C, 131, 135, 139, 186–87,
    196, 206, 231
vitamin D, 187–88, 206
vitamin E, 130, 132, 141, 186, 191,
    206, 231
vitamin K, 136, 206

walnuts, 141, 219, 238
water, 137, 214, 236
watermelon, 130, 132, 140
weight, body, 34–35, 36, 50,
    93–94, 122
whey, 26–27, 62, 126
whole foods, 115, 118, 120, 121,
    185, 208
wild rice, 217, 218
wine, 138, 216
wrinkles, reducing, 177

xylitol, 59

Yersinia pestis, 91
yoga, 42, 150, 220, 223
yogurt, 104, 127
    Greek-style, 138, 216, 218
    masks with, 174, 245
    as not triggering acne, 127
    probiotics in, 134, 138, 193,
        209

zinc, 132, 190, 206
zucchini, 242

About the Author

Renowned New York–based dermatologist Dr. Whitney Bowe has dedicated her life's work to uncovering the secrets behind glowing, healthy skin from the inside out and the outside in. A thought leader in her field and one of the most in-demand dermatologists in the country, Dr. Bowe has earned the attention of top media outlets, netting her invitations to share her expertise on television programs such as *Good Morning America, The Rachael Ray Show, The Doctors,* and *The Dr. Oz Show* and in publications such as the *Wall Street Journal,* the *New York Times, Allure,* and *InStyle.*

Always with her finger on the pulse of the latest research, technological developments, and product and treatment trends, Dr. Bowe maintains an easy, accessible approach to explaining even the most complex medical terminology and concepts, an approach that has truly established her as America's dermatologist.

Dr. Bowe attended Yale University, from which she graduated summa cum laude with a bachelor of science degree in molecular, cellular, and developmental biology. Subsequently she was awarded a full scholarship to study medicine at the University of Pennsylvania, from which she graduated at the top of her class.

Medical director of integrative dermatology, aesthetics, and wellness at Advanced Dermatology, PC, Dr. Bowe uses cutting-edge technology and injection techniques to achieve her signature ageless aesthetic, which she refers to as the New Natural. Dr. Bowe also serves as the clinical assistant professor of dermatology at the Icahn School of Medicine at Mount Sinai, in New York City. Her outstanding research in microbiology has earned her scores of awards from renowned organizations such as the Skin Cancer Foundation and has earned her invitations to make presentations at numerous international conferences each year.

Named to a coveted position on the *Super Doctors* list, Dr. Bowe holds a patent for a bacterium-derived acne treatment. She has written more than forty articles and book chapters and has conducted clinical trials that explore new forms of treatment for acne. She also serves as a consultant and trusted adviser to numerous national and global companies, helping in the development and evaluation of novel topical and ingestible products.

In her free time, Dr. Bowe loves spending time outdoors with her daughter, Maclane, and husband of fourteen years, Josh. Dr. Bowe fuels her inner and outer glow with the things that make her happiest and most inspired and, above all else, spark her signature #boweglow.